VETERINARY
OPHTHALMOLOGY

VETERINARY OPHTHALMOLOGY

KEITH C BARNETT
OBE MA PhD BSc DVOphthal FRCVS DipECVO RCVS

Specialist in Veterinary Ophthalmology
Head of Centre for Small Animal Studies
Animal Health Trust
Lanwades Park
Kennett
Near Newmarket

Associate Lecturer
Department of Clinical Veterinary Medicine
University of Cambridge

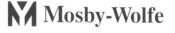 Mosby-Wolfe

London Baltimore Barcelona Bogotá Boston Buenos Aires Carlsbad, CA Chicago Madrid Mexico City Milan Naples, FL New York
Philadelphia St. Louis Seoul Singapore Sydney Taipei Tokyo Toronto Wiesbaden

Copyright © K C Barnett, 1990

Published by Mosby-Wolfe, an imprint of Times Mirror International Publishers Ltd.

Reprinted in 1996

ISBN 0 7234 1504 8 (Cased edition)

ISBN 0 7234 2956 1 (Limp edition)

A CIP catalogue record for this book is available from the British Library.

For full details of all Times Mirror International Publishers Limited titles please write to Times Mirror International Publishers Limited, Lynton House, 7–12 Tavistock Square, London WC1H 9LB, England.

Contents

Acknowledgements

I wish to acknowledge the interest of the veterinary surgeons who referred all the animals depicted in this book, the co-operation of their owners and breeders and, most particularly, the animals themselves whose patience enabled me to photograph their eye problems. I also acknowledge the assistance and encouragement of my staff and colleagues at both Cambridge and Newmarket.

This Atlas is in memory of M.G. (Will) Thomas who, although only recently qualified, was already showing a great interest in veterinary ophthalmology before he sadly died.

Preface

This book is intended both for the practising veterinary surgeon and also for the student with an interest in eye diseases. It is designed to complement existing textbooks of veterinary ophthalmology and provides a valuable pictorial resource for any clinician working in this field.

Special emphasis is given to the dog, cat and horse, with additional material on cattle and sheep. The subject matter covered is, however, relevant to a wide variety of species. Full-colour photographs are used to illustrate the appearance and progression of a range of eye diseases, featuring the essential presenting signs to aid the user in making a more accurate diagnosis. A comprehensive supporting text highlights differences in the incidence of particular disorders in relation to breed, and to age within breed.

The Colour Atlas of Veterinary Ophthalmology will be useful to final year veterinary students and to qualified veterinary surgeons worldwide who are studying for specialist qualifications such as the Certificate and Diploma in Veterinary Ophthalmology of the Royal College of Veterinary Surgeons, the Diploma of the American College of Veterinary Ophthalmologists, and their equivalents.

The Globe

This first section covers the eye as a whole, whereas following sections deal with specific parts of the globe, e.g. cornea, lens, retina, etc. A degree of overlap between this section and those that follow is, therefore, inevitable and certain illustrations used in this treatment of the globe could have appeared elsewhere, e.g. microcornea, episcleritis and dermoids.

Prior to detailed examination of parts of the eye it is advisable to make a naked-eye examination of the eye as a whole, perhaps assisted with a simple pen torch, and assess ocular movements. At this initial examination the size of the globe and its position within the orbit should be noted and any discrepancies recorded. Prominence or degrees of enophthalmos, together with the position of the nictitating membrane, may all be vital in reaching an accurate diagnosis.

The normal eye (1) should be compared with the series on exophthalmos (6 to 9), hydrophthalmos (10), eyeball prolapse (2) and the series on microphthalmos (11 to 14), phthisis bulbi (15) and microcornea (16).

The section concludes with a series of photographs of neuro-ophthalmological conditions. These are particularly difficult to illustrate in an atlas of this type and the series is not intended to be comprehensive.

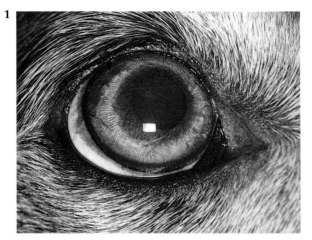

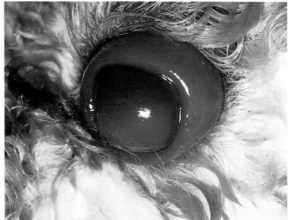

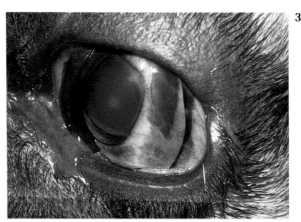

1 **The normal eye (Greyhound, young adult)** Note the shape and perfect apposition of the eyelids to the globe, the absence of any discharge, and the regular corneal reflection.

2 **Eyeball prolapse (Miniature Poodle, young adult)** Following trauma the globe is trapped in front of the eyelids and thereby prevented from returning to the orbit. Note intraocular and subconjunctival haemorrhage, not present in all cases of globe prolapse.

3 **Bruising and subconjunctival haemorrhage (Crossbred adult)** The result of various types of injury in all species. These changes are transient and will leave no permanent abnormality.

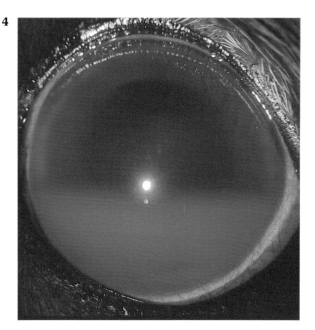

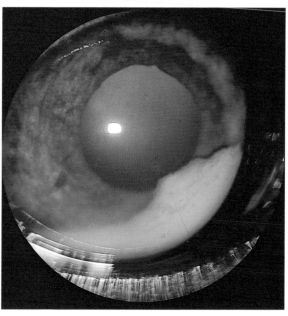

4 Hyphaema (Chihuahua, 7 years old) Blood in the anterior chamber. Differential diagnoses: trauma, tumour, collie eye anomaly (*see* **531**), clotting abnormality e.g. thrombocytopaenia, as in this case.

5 Hypopyon (Boxer, adult) Pus in the anterior chamber - usually associated with iritis.

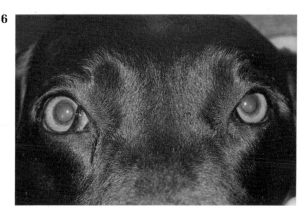

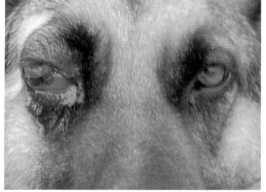

6 Exophthalmos or proptosis (Labrador, 8 years old) Note the prominence of the globe and the nictitating membrane, changed shape of the palpebral orifice and epiphora of the right eye. The retrobulbar mass proved to be a glioma of the optic nerve closely applied to the back of the globe and was also the cause of a retinal detachment.

7 Exophthalmos (German Shepherd Dog, 3 years old) Note the obvious prominence of the globe, again with prominence of the third eyelid, and periorbital swelling. The retrobulbar mass proved to be a spindle cell sarcoma.

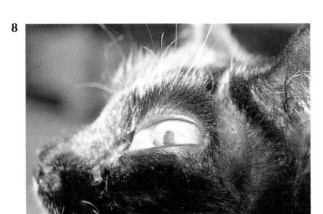

8 Exophthalmos (DSH cat, 9 years old) Prominence of the globe and nictitating membrane, with periorbital swelling and change in the palpebral aperture, due to a retrobulbar lymphosarcoma.

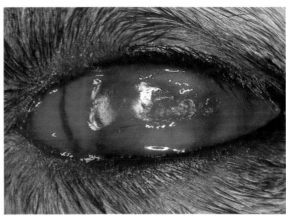

9 Exophthalmos (Greyhound, young adult) Prominence of the globe and third eyelid with central exposure keratitis and ocular discharge. This acute case of exophthalmos was accompanied by pain and was due to a retrobulbar abscess.

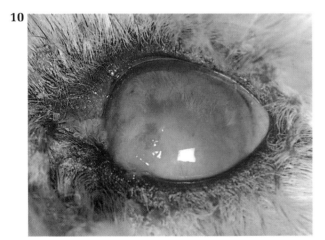

10 Hydrophthalmos (Sealyham, 6 years old) Relative oversize of the globe due to a secondary and uncontrolled glaucoma, the primary condition in this case being lens luxation. Note the retraction of the nictitating membrane in comparison to the previous cases of exophthalmos in which the globe is of normal size (*see also* buphthalmos, **247**).

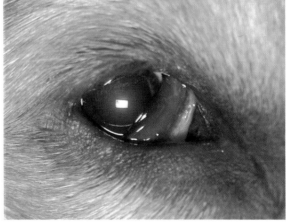

11 Microphthalmos (Rough Collie, young adult) A small eye with no other ocular anomaly. Congenital and may be considered normal in certain breeds. Note the prominence of the nictitating membrane accompanying the small and sunken globe (*see also* **283–296**).

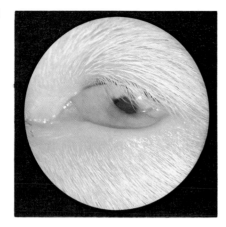

12 Microphthalmos (Shetland Sheepdog, 7 weeks old, white) Severe microphthalmos and deafness, the result of a blue merle x blue merle mating.

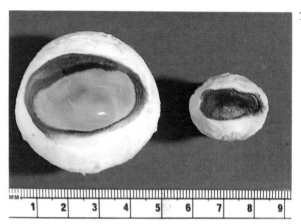

13 Microphthalmos (Thoroughbred foal) Known as 'button eye' in the horse. The condition is congenital and occurs in all breeds of horse but particularly the Thoroughbred. It is often accompanied by multiple congenital anomalies, as in this case. The photograph shows differing degrees in the two eyes of the same foal, other cases may show only one eye apparently affected.

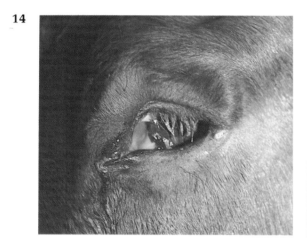

14 Phthisis bulbi (Polo pony) Shrivelled and sunken globe, again with prominence of the third eyelid. This condition occurs in all species but more commonly in the horse. It follows severe trauma, intraocular infection or inflammation and glaucoma. *See also* **346**.

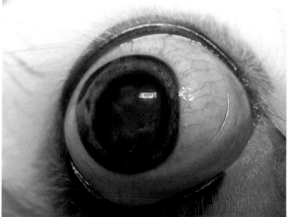

15 Microcornea (Old English Sheepdog, 3 months old) Normal-sized globe but small corneal diameter, together with other ocular abnormalities. Congenital.

16 Epibulbar dermoid (German Shepherd Dog, 3 months old) Congenital, commonly pigmented and hairy and typically affecting the cornea and adjacent limbus at the lateral canthus.

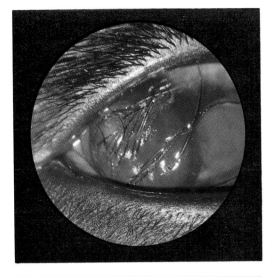

17 Epibulbar dermoid (German Shepherd Dog, 5 weeks old) In this case mainly affecting the palpebral conjunctiva at the lateral canthus. Note also a deficiency of the eyelid edge at the canthus.

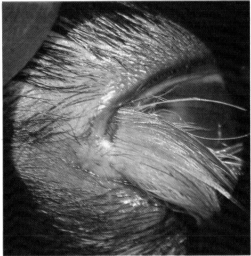

18 Epibulbar dermoid (Thoroughbred foal) A pigmented non-hairy and cystic dermoid at the superior limbus. Note also corneal opacity. Dermoids in the horse are usually seen at the limbus and rarely cause any problem.

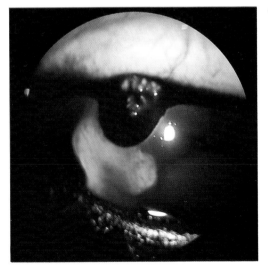

19

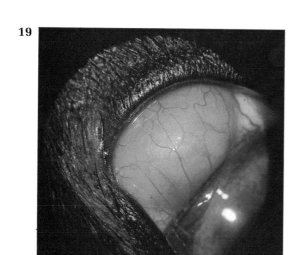

19 Episcleritis or nodular fasciitis (Border Collie, 3 years old) A slowly-developing, pinkish-cream, subconjunctival mass usually occurring on the sclera. Characterised histologically by inflammatory rather than neoplastic cells.

20

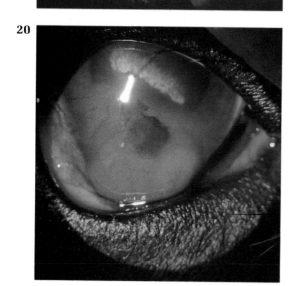

20 Episcleritis or nodular fasciitis (Miniature Wire-haired Dachshund, 3 years old) In this case the lesion has infiltrated into the cornea. Note the vascularisation and pigmentation and the area of lipid keratopathy superior to the swelling.

21

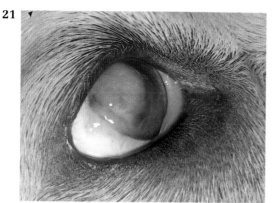

21 Episcleritis or nodular fasciitis (Rough Collie, 4 years old) A typical case in this breed and sometimes referred to as proliferative keratoconjunctivitis.

22 Squamous cell carcinoma of the globe (Hereford adult cow) This malignant neoplasm originally affects part of the globe e.g. conjunctiva, cornea, limbus, nictitating membrane. *See* **67–68, 97, 112–114** and **177–178**.

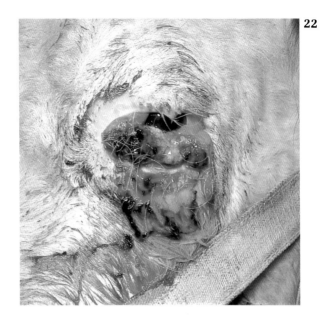

23 Strabismus (Boxer, 9 weeks old) Marked squint following trauma and prolapse of the globe.

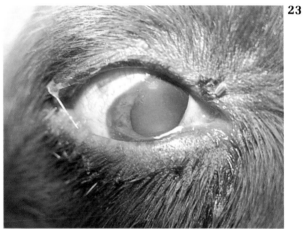

24 Strabismus (English Springer Spaniel, 2 years old) Divergent squint associated with a retrobulbar tumour (adenocarcinoma).

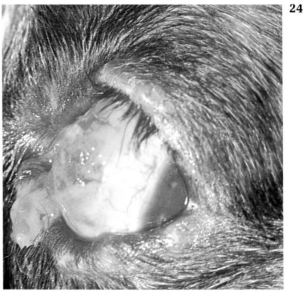

25 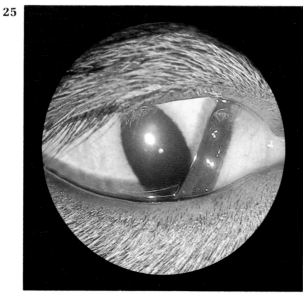 **26**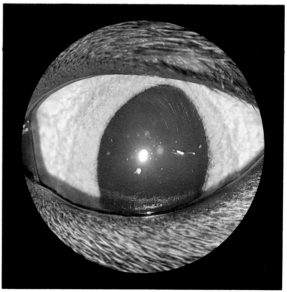

27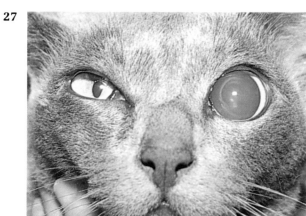

25 and 26 Horner's syndrome (DSH cat, adult) A normal left eye, with an affected right eye showing the classical signs of ptosis of the upper lid, producing a different shape of palpebral orifice, enophthalmos with consequent prominence of the third eyelid and miosis. This cat had a concurrent otitis media.

27 Anisocoria (Burmese cat, 4 years old) The pupils are of unequal size, dilated on the left side with the absence of a pupillary light reflex. Unknown aetiology.

28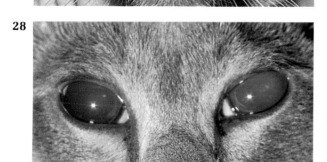

28 Feline dysautonomia or Key-Gaskell Syndrome (Burmese kitten) Note the total dilation of both pupils, with absence of the pupillary light reflex and prominence of the nictitating membranes.

The Eyelids

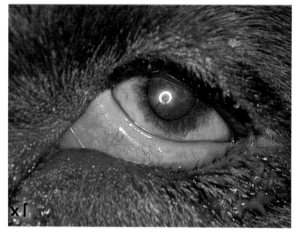

This section illustrates the many and varied forms of entropion, both hereditary (**29** to **37**) and non-hereditary (**39**), and shows the various types of abnormality associated with different breeds. The breed incidence and age incidence within each breed are demonstrated, as well as eye shape, excessive facial skin and nasal folds, all of which materially affect this condition. The section also illustrates ectropion (**41** to **44**), which is much less common than entropion, but is again associated with eye shape and has a characteristic breed incidence.

Other eyelid conditions, undoubtedly associated with a hereditary factor and extremely common in the dog, are distichiasis, ectopic cilia and trichiasis. All three fall within the category of supernumerary eyelashes and are of variable clinical importance.

Inflammation of the eyelids and congenital abnormalities are shown, together with several types of eyelid tumours. These are particularly common in ageing animals and are illustrated in the dog, cat and horse. Note the appearance of the tumour in relation to the histopathological diagnosis given under each figure.

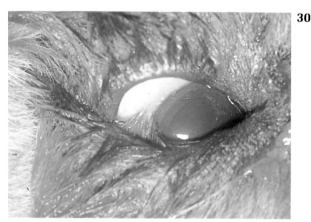

29 Entropion (German Short-haired Pointer, 14 weeks old) In-turned lower lid causing irritation and consequent enophthalmos with prominence of the nictitating membrane.

30 Entropion (Chow, 8 months old) Hairs of the face causing irritation and profuse lacrimation.

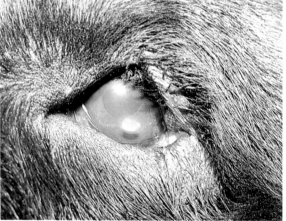

31 Entropion (Rottweiler, 4 years old) Typical lower lid entropion together with upper lid involvement. In this breed the condition often occurs in adult dogs. Compare the age in this breed with those in **29** and **30, 32** and **33**.

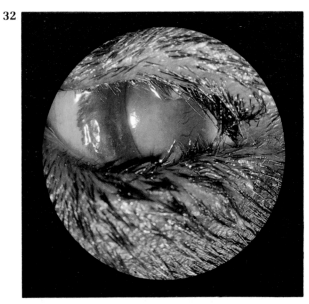

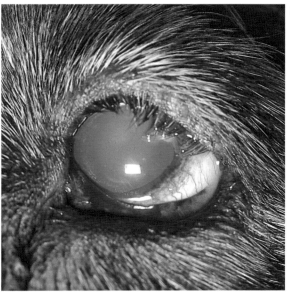

32 Entropion (Great Dane, 7 weeks old) Upper and lower lid entropion with corneal vascularisation.

33 Entropion (Cocker Spaniel, 10 years old) Senile entropion of the upper lid. Occurs typically in this breed.

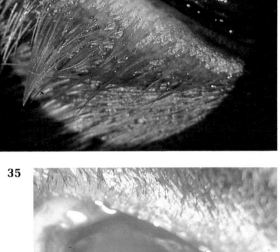

34 Entropion (Golden Retriever, 8 months old) Typical sign of depigmentation where the eyelid edge has been rolled inwards and come in contact with the tear film.

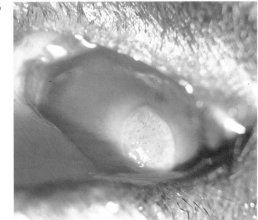

35 Entropion (Chow, 13 months old) Corneal granulation tissue resulting from chronic irritation.

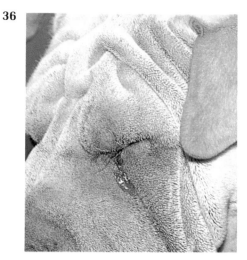

36 Entropion (Shar Pei, 12 months old) Entropion associated with multiple facial folds. Note the closed eye.

37 Entropion (Shar Pei, 12 months old) Granulation tissue, corneal scarring and altered pigmentation due to severe irritation from facial hairs.

38 Entropion (Pekingese, 4 years old) Entropion and corneal ulcer associated with a nasal fold.

39 Entropion (Pembroke Corgi, 6 weeks old) Traumatic entropion following a split eyelid.

40 Entropion (Dorset Horn, 3 days old) Entropion in the sheep, and in the Thoroughbred, is often both congenital and hereditary.

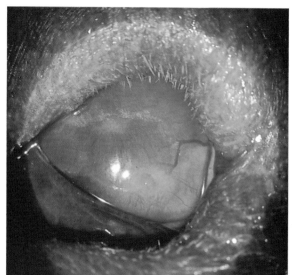

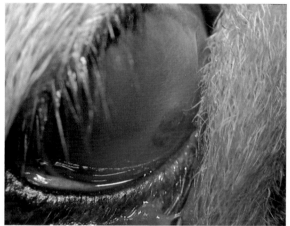

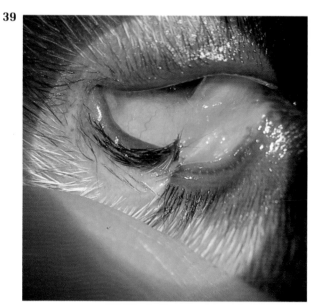

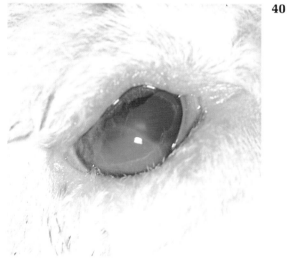

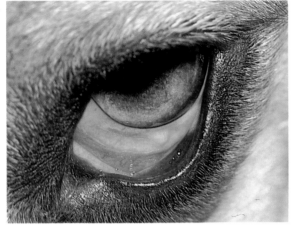

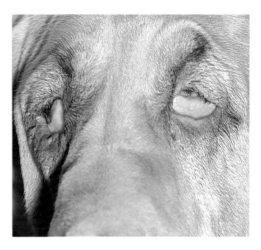

41 Ectropion (Beagle, young adult) Slack lower lid due to too long a lid.

42 Ectropion (Bloodhound, young adult) Enophthalmos, prominence of the nictitating membranes (haw) and ectropion of the lower lids, sometimes complicated by entropion of the upper lids and due to excessive skin on the head.

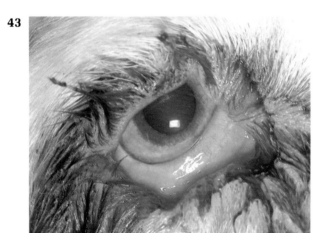

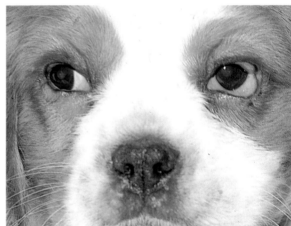

43 Ectropion (Clumber Spaniel, young adult) The diamond eye with ectropion at the kink in the centre of the lid, sometimes complicated by entropion on either side.

44 Ectropion (Cavalier King Charles Spaniel puppy) Ectropion of both upper and lower lids with eyelid-swelling due to juvenile pyoderma. Note also the affected muzzle.

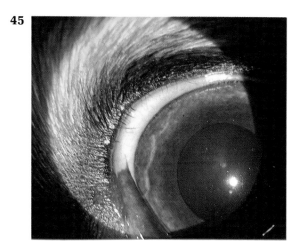

45 Distichiasis (Miniature Long-haired Dachshund, 1 year old) Very common in this breed.

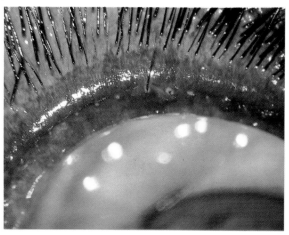

46 Distichiasis (Flat-coated Retriever, 2 years old) Two supernumerary cilia arising from the meibomian gland opening.

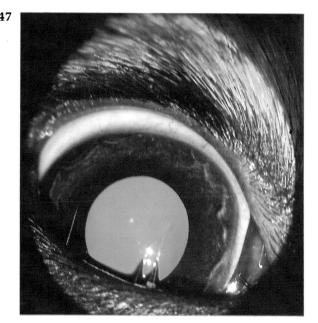

47 Distichiasis (Miniature Long-haired Dachshund, young adult) Note the long supernumerary cilia producing slight excess in tear production but no corneal damage.

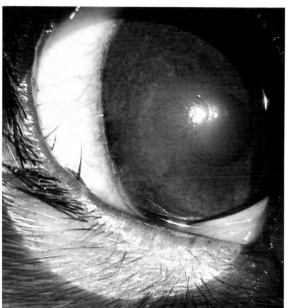

48 Distichiasis (Pekingese, young adult) Short cilia causing corneal ulcer.

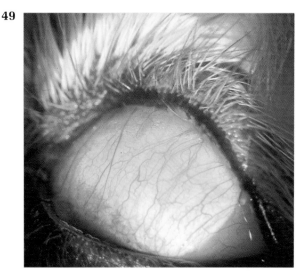

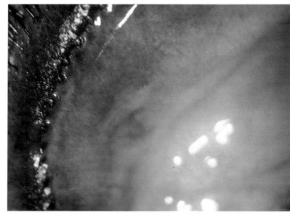

49 Distichiasis and ectopic cilia (Pekingese, 1 year old) Ectopic cilia are invariably found together with distichiasis.

50 Ectopic cilia (Flat-coated Retriever, 7 months old) Note the origin of aberrant cilia well inside the upper eyelid margin.

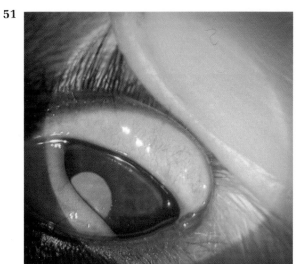

51 Ectopic cilia (Shetland Sheepdog, 4 months old) Several potential ectopic cilia still beneath the palpebral conjunctiva.

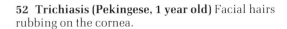
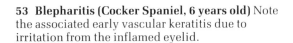

52 Trichiasis (Pekingese, 1 year old) Facial hairs rubbing on the cornea.

53 Blepharitis (Cocker Spaniel, 6 years old) Note the associated early vascular keratitis due to irritation from the inflamed eyelid.

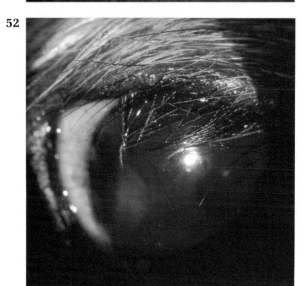

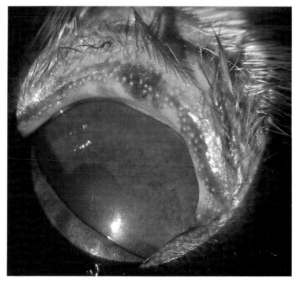

54

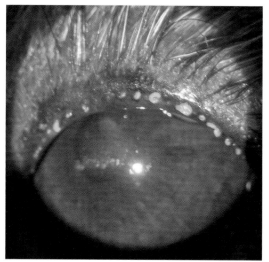

54 Meibomitis (Cavalier King Charles Spaniel, 4 years old) Note the secretion from the glands.

55 Chalazion (Labrador, 8 weeks old) Infected and distended meibomian glands.

56 Meibomian cyst (Beagle, young adult) Cystic distension on the conjunctival side of the lid.

57 Agenesis or eyelid coloboma (DSH cat, 1 year old) Congenital absence of the outer half of both upper eyelids.

58 Coloboma of eyelid (Staffordshire Bull Terrier, 2 weeks old) Congenital lower lid coloboma and corneal ulcer. Rare.

55

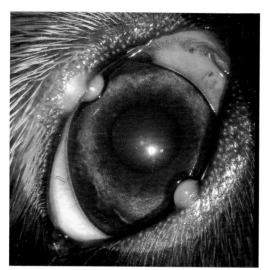

56

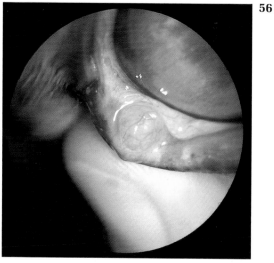

57

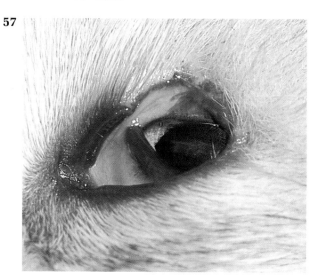

58

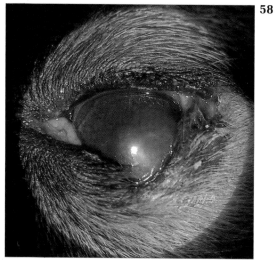

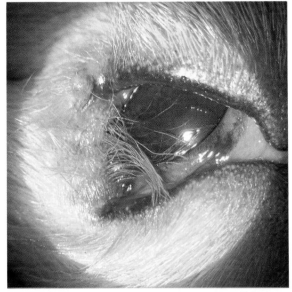

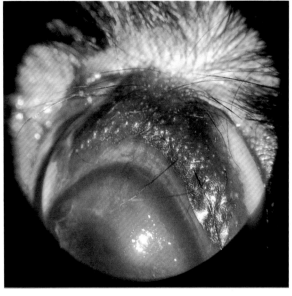

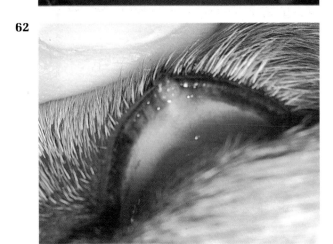

59 Eyelid deformity (Labrador, 6 weeks old) Gross congenital deformity of the eyelids.

60 Eyelid deformity (Shih Tzu puppy) Congenital deformity of the eyelid with dermoid.

61 Eyelid tumour—papilloma (Irish Setter, 7 years old)

62 Eyelid tumour—papilloma (Pembroke Corgi, 9 years old) Note extension into the substance of the lid visible on palpebral surface.

63 Eyelid tumour—squamous papilloma (Labrador, 9 years old)

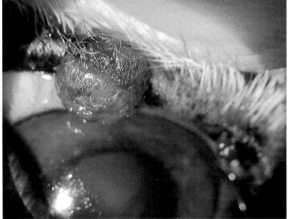

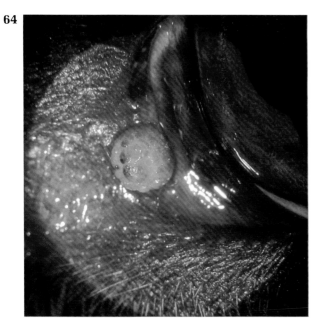

64 Eyelid tumour—viral papilloma (Golden Retriever, 1 year old)

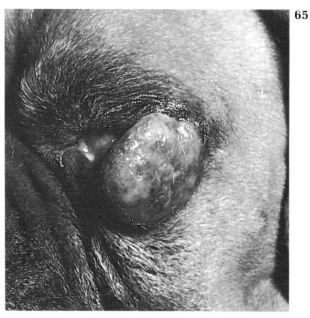

65 Eyelid tumour—mast cell tumour (Boxer, 9 years old)

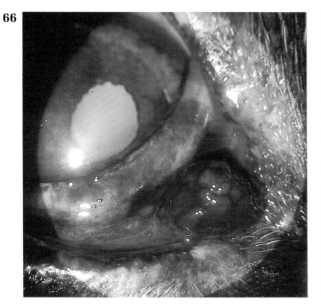

66 Eyelid tumour—melanoma (Beagle, 10 years old)

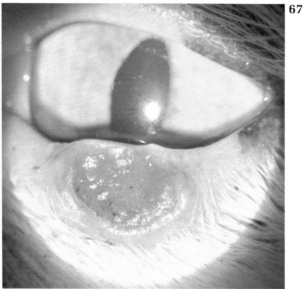

67 Eyelid tumour—squamous cell carcinoma (Tabby/white DSH cat, 12 years old)

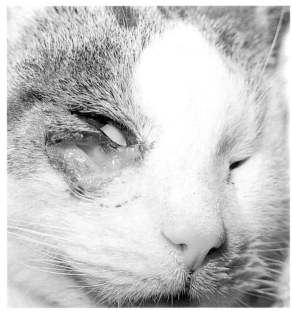

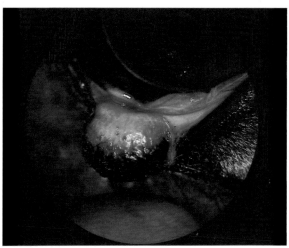

69 Eyelid tumour—sarcoid (New Forest Pony mare, 13 years old)

68 Eyelid tumour—squamous cell carcinoma (Tabby/white DSH cat, 14 years old)

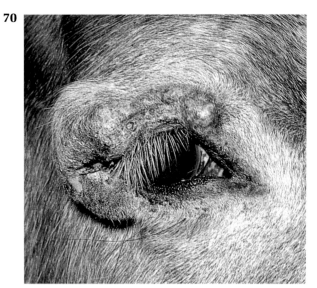

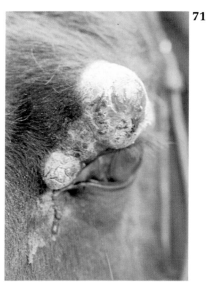

70 Eyelid tumour—sarcoid (Welsh Pony gelding, 8 years old)

71 Eyelid tumour—sarcoid (Welsh Cob stallion, 5 years old)

The Nasolacrimal Duct System

A wet eye is often a presenting sign to the veterinary surgeon and the differential diagnosis should first investigate as to whether the condition is due to lacrimation (increased tear production) or epiphora (decreased tear drainage).

Micro and imperforate puncta are inherited in some breeds, for example the Cocker Spaniel and Golden Retriever (**73** and **74**), but can also be due to trauma (**77**). Blockage of the nasolacrimal duct, and consequent epiphora, can also be due to infection and/or foreign body.

In this section the appearance of the normal punctum is compared with the congenital conditions of micropunctum and imperforate punctum. Other conditions illustrated include occlusion of the punctum due to trauma, nasolacrimal duct infection and foreign body.

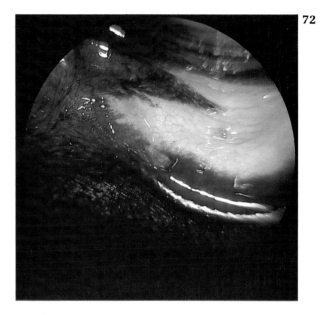

72 The normal punctum—lower eyelid

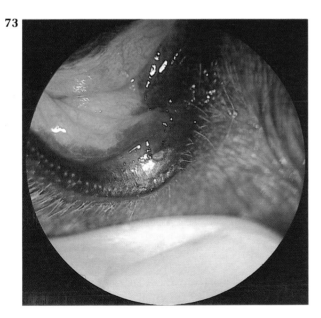

73 Micropunctum (Cocker Spaniel, 8 months old)
Note the thickened edge of the opening.

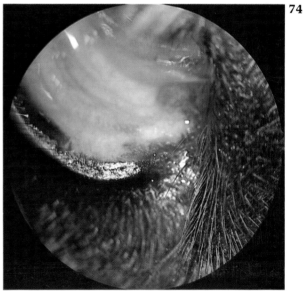

74 Imperforate punctum (Golden Retriever, 6 months old)

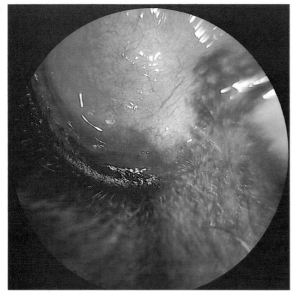 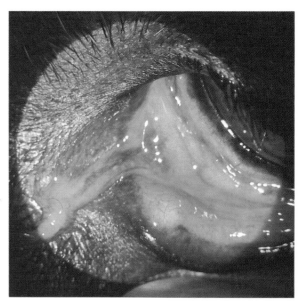

75 Imperforate punctum (Basset Hound, 14 months old) Note the depression over the position of the duct.

76 Imperforate punctum (Wire-haired Dachshund, 5 years old) Note the purulent discharge and abscess at the blind end of the duct.

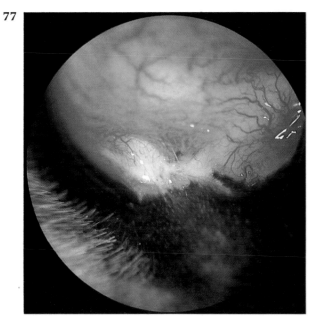 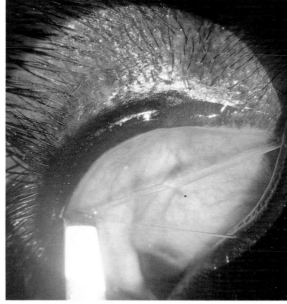

77 Occluded punctum (Crossbred terrier, 6 months old) Traumatic origin.

78 Nasolacrimal duct infection (Crossbred, 10 months old) Mucus strand from the lower punctum following irrigation via the upper punctum.

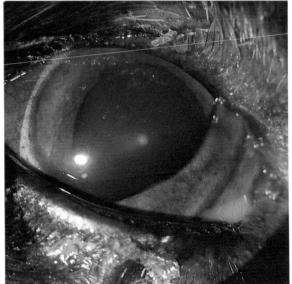

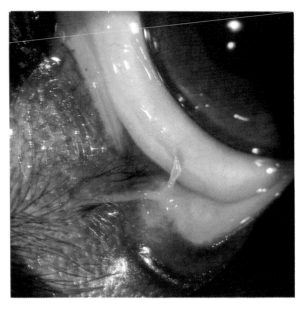

79 Nasolacrimal duct infection (Rough Collie, 6 years old) Note the persistent and purulent ocular discharge and the bead of pus at the inner canthus.

80 Nasolacrimal duct foreign body (Old English Sheepdog, 14 months old) Grass awn protruding from the lower punctum following irrigation via the upper punctum.

81 Tear streak (Golden Retriever, 6 months old) Note the typical appearance of a brown stain from the inner canthus in a case of imperforate punctum.

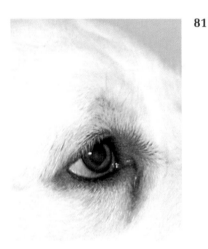

82 Imperforate punctum (Thoroughbred foal, 8 months old) Note the purulent ocular discharge—the usual clinical sign in the horse where this defect occurs commonly at the nasal punctum.

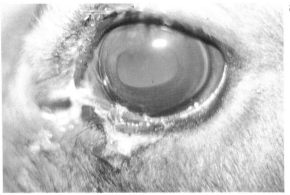

The Nictitating Membrane

83

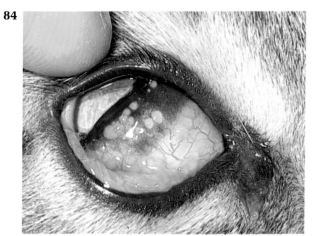

The nictitating membrane, or third eyelid (haw), is covered with palpebral conjunctiva, as are the eyelids, and can therefore show conjunctival conditions such as inflammation, oedema, etc. The prominence, or otherwise, of the nictitating membrane relates to the position of the globe and these conditions have been illustrated in the first section, 'The Globe'.

Deformity of the cartilage of the third eyelid is an important and not uncommon condition seen particularly in the larger dog breeds. It must be distinguished from prolapse of the nictitans gland as well as from various tumours of the membrane and its gland.

Inflammation, oedema, cyst and various deformities of the cartilage are shown, together with gland prolapse, granuloma and tumours.

83 Follicular conjunctivitis (English Springer Spaniel, 14 months old) This condition particularly affects both aspects of the nictitating membrane and other palpebral conjunctiva.

84

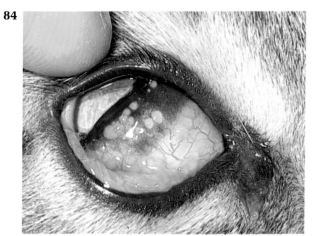

85

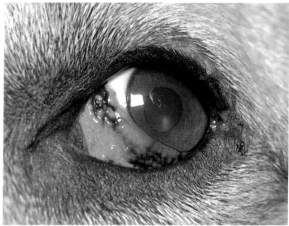

84 Follicular conjunctivitis (DSH cat, 12 months old) Note the depigmentation in the region of the follicles and serous ocular discharge.

85 Plasma cell infiltration (German Shepherd Dog, 7 years old) Again note depigmentation of the affected region. This condition frequently accompanies pannus (see **125-127**)

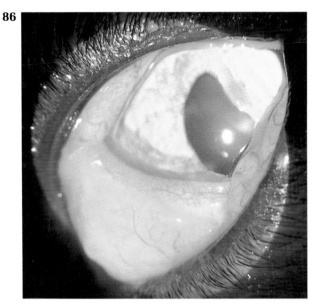

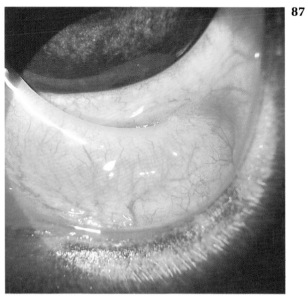

86 Chemosis (DSH cat, 11 years old) Bulbar and palpebral conjunctiva affected. *See also* **100**.

87 Conjunctival cyst (English Setter, 8 months old) Cyst at the base of the third eyelid. *See also* **105** and **106**.

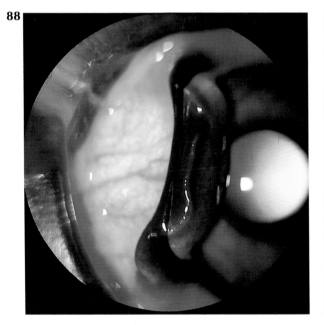

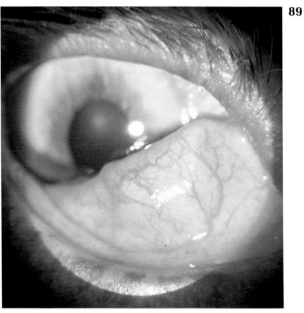

88 Cartilage deformity (German Shepherd Dog, 7 months old) Free border of the third eyelid rolled outwards.

89 Cartilage deformity (Weimaraner, 5 years old) Free border of cartilage rolled inwards.

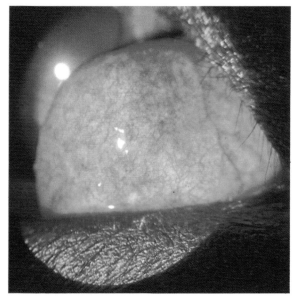

90 Cartilage deformity (Great Dane, 8 months old)
As **89.** A differential diagnosis with prolapsed
nictitans gland (*see* **91**).

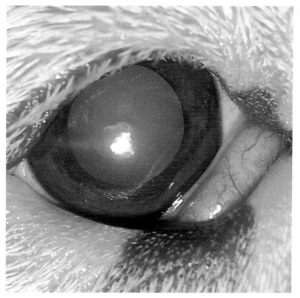

**91 Prolapse of the nictitans gland (Bulldog, 2 years
old)** Note the visible free border of the nictitating
membrane (not apparent in the previous two
figures).

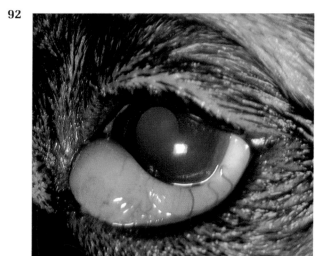

**92 Prolapse of the nictitans gland (Bulldog, 10
weeks old)** This breed is particularly prone to this
condition.

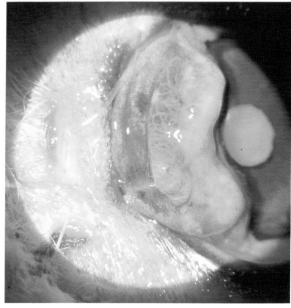

**93 Prolapse of the nictitans gland (Miniature
Poodle, 4 years old)** Torn and prolapsed nictitans
gland and third eyelid following trauma.

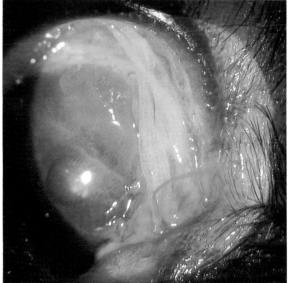

94 Nictitating membrane foreign body (Tibetan Terrier, 2 years old) Grass awn behind the third eyelid. Note the corneal granulation tissue.

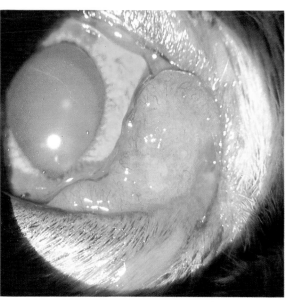

95 Granuloma of the nictitating membrane (Persian cat, 18 months old) The condition was bilateral and of unknown aetiology.

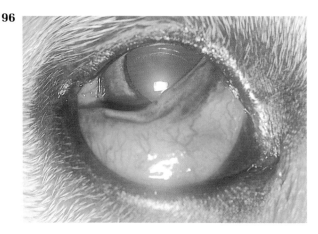

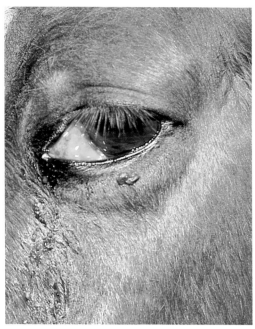

96 Nictitating membrane tumour—lymphosarcoma (Labrador, 3 years old) Tumours of the third eyelid are rare in the dog.

97 Nictitating membrane tumour—squamous cell carcinoma (horse, 8 years old) A common site for this type of tumour in the horse.

The Conjunctiva

Conjunctivitis of the bulbar conjunctiva is probably the most obvious and common eye condition, occurring in all animals. It is of very varied aetiology and only a few examples are illustrated here. Congestion of the conjunctival blood vessels may also be associated with pyrexia and systemic disease, for example canine distemper and equine influenza. Symblepharon, or adhesion of conjunctiva to cornea which is typically seen in the cat, is the result of such a conjunctivitis associated with upper respiratory tract infections.

Inflammation, oedema, haemorrhage, deposits, foreign body and cysts are illustrated, together with symblepharon of varying degrees of severity and conjuctival tumours in the horse, dog and cat.

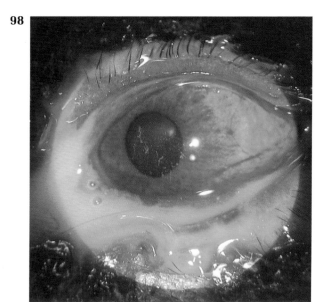

98 Purulent conjunctivitis (Long-haired Dachshund, 9 months old) Note that the discharge is not adherent to the cornea, as it is in cases of keratoconjunctivitis sicca (*see* **147**).

99 Follicular conjunctivitis (Balinese cat, 2 years old) Note some chemosis and ocular discharge. *See also* **83** and **84**.

100 Conjunctival oedema or chemosis (DSH cat, 3 years old) Positive for chlamydia.

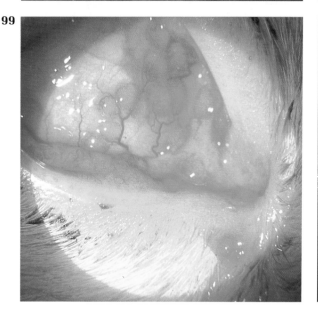

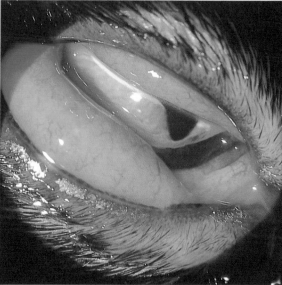

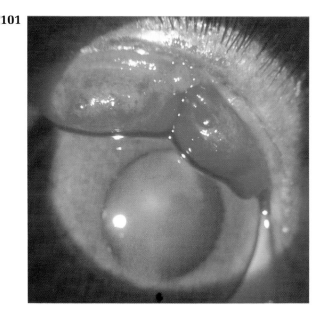

101 Subconjunctival haemorrhage (English Springer Spaniel, 10 years old) This particular case was a reaction to paint stripper.

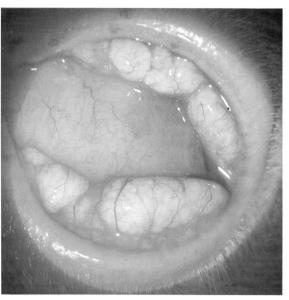

102 Subconjunctival masses (Burmese cat, 9 years old) An inflammatory deposit beneath the palpebral conjunctiva. Both eyes affected, unknown aetiology.

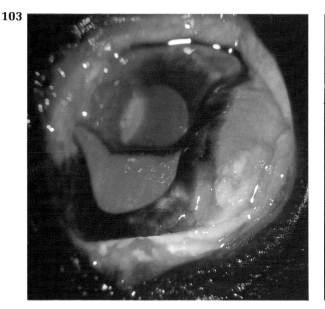

103 Conjunctival calcinosis (Munsterlander, 5 months old) In this case the outer aspect of the nictitating membrane and bulbar conjunctiva are affected. Note also the condition of the nictitating membrane, the vascular keratitis and corneal ulcer.

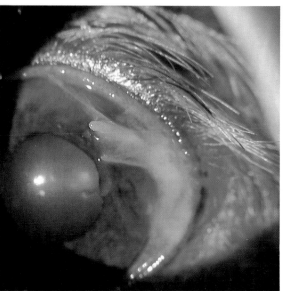

104 Conjunctival foreign body (Yorkshire Terrier, 8 years old) Grass awn in the upper lateral conjunctival fornix. *See also* **94**.

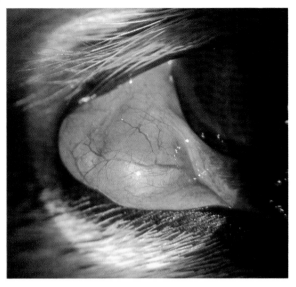

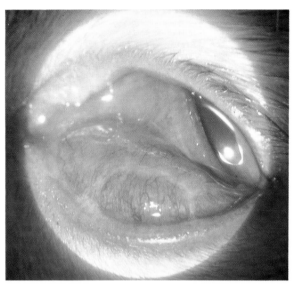

105 Conjunctival cyst (Golden Retriever, 6 months old) *See also* **87**.

106 Conjunctival cyst (Siamese cat, 10 months old) Rare in this species.

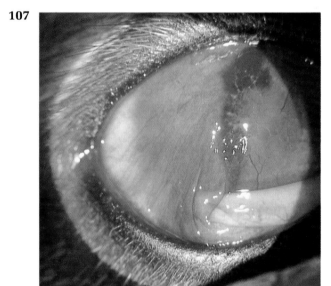

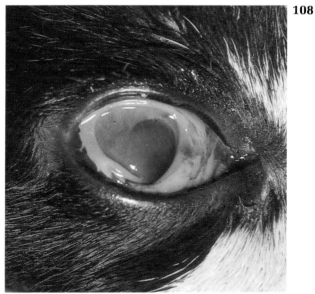

107 Symblepharon (Cavalier King Charles Spaniel, 15 weeks old) Congenital adhesion of the palpebral conjunctiva to the cornea. Rare in this species.

108 Symblepharon (DSH cat, 2 years old) Adhesion of the palpebral conjunctiva to the cornea obliterating the conjunctival fornices. Relatively common in this species.

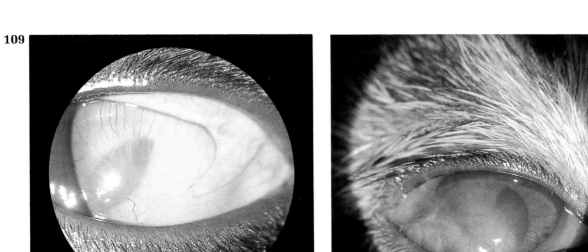

109 Symblepharon (DSH cat, 6 months old)

110 Symblepharon (DSH cat, 5 weeks old) An early case. Ocular discharge was noted as early as 10 days of age.

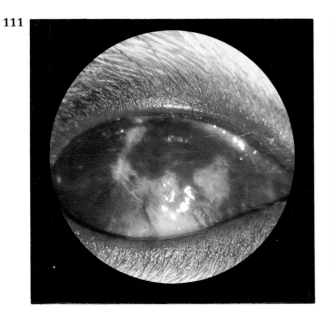

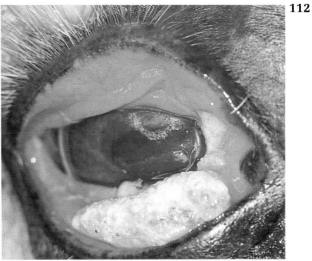

112 Conjunctival tumour—squamous cell carcinoma (Palomino hunter, 13 years old) Lower palpebral conjunctiva and nictitating membrane.

111 Symblepharon (DSH cat, 7 months old) A very severe case.

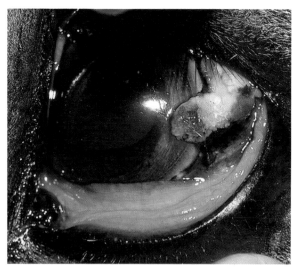

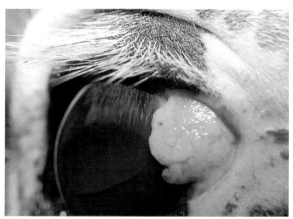

114 Conjunctival tumour—squamous cell carcinoma (Hunter gelding, 17 years old) Similar position to the previous figure.

113 Conjunctival tumour—squamous cell carcinoma (Connemara pony, 8 years old) Bulbar conjunctiva at the limbus.

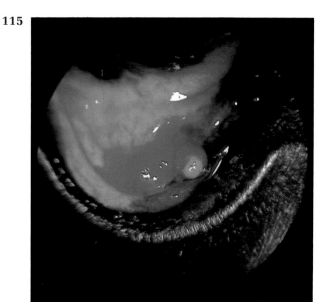

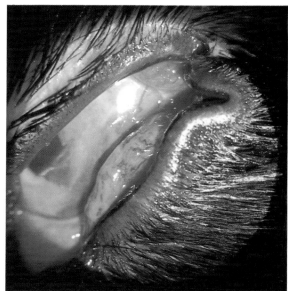

115 Conjunctival tumour—benign haemangioma (Gordon Setter, 11 years old) Lower conjunctival fornix.

116 Conjunctival tumour—lymphosarcoma (DSH cat, 11 years old) Palpebral conjunctiva and nictitating membrane.

The Cornea

Keratitis is another common eye condition in all species and again has many causes. The extension of inflammation between cornea and conjunctiva, which results in the condition of keratoconjunctivitis, leads to some overlap with the previous section. This large section covers the varying forms of keratitis in a number of species, some specific, others not.

Vascular keratitis or pannus, for instance, is seen typically in the German Shepherd Dog. The clinical signs characteristic of keratoconjunctivitis sicca or dry eye, are all illustrated. The corneal ulcer is a common and sometimes difficult eye condition in small animals and several forms of corneal ulcer of varying degrees of severity are shown. Corneal oedema presents as a corneal opacity and its

appearance in the dog, horse and calf is illustrated.

Trauma, including abscess, rupture and foreign body are illustrated as well as the congenital condition of corneal dermoid. Three cases of corneal sequestrum, a condition unique to the cat, depict different degrees of this condition.

Lipid keratopathies again present as corneal opacities and occur particularly in the dog. They can be subdivided into corneal lipidosis, corneal dystrophy and corneal degeneration, each occurring in particular breeds, and other lipid keratopathies associated with different ocular anomalies.

Corneal tumours are rare but two examples of carcinoma in the horse are included.

117

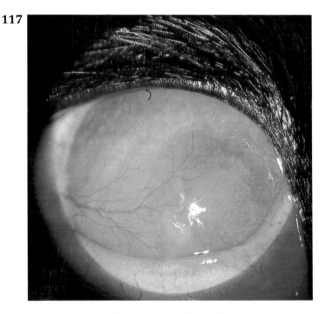

118

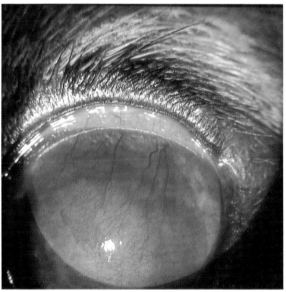

117 Superficial keratitis (Border Collie, 9 years old) Note the blood vessel crossing the limbus and the irregular corneal surface (with break up of corneal reflection).

118 Interstitial keratitis (Miniature Wire-haired Dachshund, 2 years old) Note the blood vessels at the limbus and typical vascular branching.

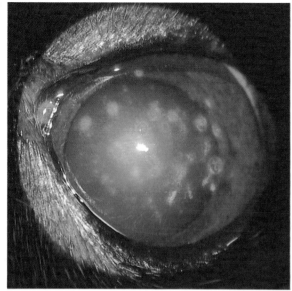

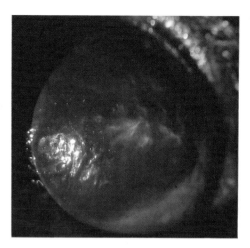

120 Pigmentary keratitis (Pug, 6 years old) May be accompanied by vascular keratitis.

119 Punctate keratitis (Shetland Sheepdog, 8 years old) Usually bilateral and the areas may take fluorescein stain.

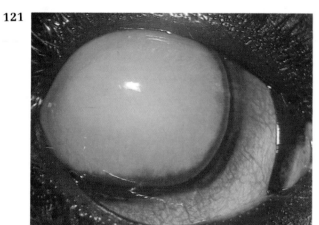

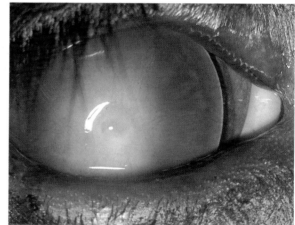

121 Infectious bovine keratoconjunctivitis (Friesian calf) Note the corneal opacity, vascular fringe and conjunctival congestion.

122 Infectious bovine keratoconjunctivitis (Friesian calf) Note the central opaque and vascularised area following ulceration.

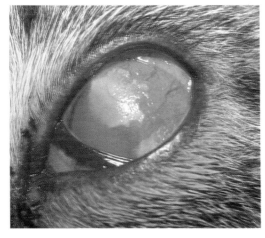

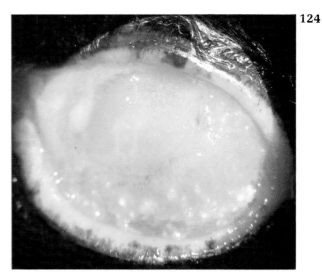

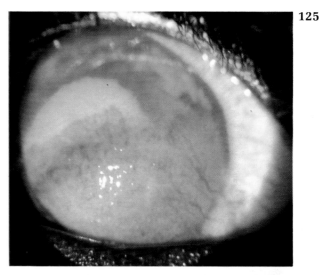

123 Eosinophilic keratitis (DSH cat, 1 year old) A unilateral case.

124 Eosinophilic keratitis (DSH cat, 3 years old) A bilateral case. Note typical white plaques.

125 Pannus (German Shepherd Dog, 4 years old) Chronic superficial vascular keratitis.

126 Pannus (German Shepherd Dog, 9 years old) Pigmentary type.

127 Pannus (German Shepherd Dog, 3 years old) Involvement of the nictitating membrane (*see also* **85**).

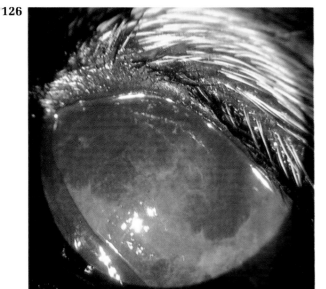

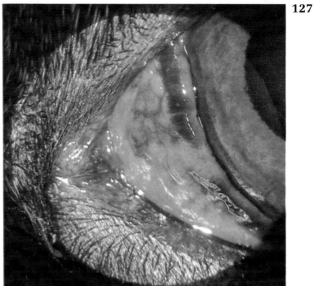

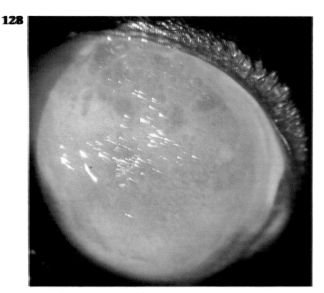

128

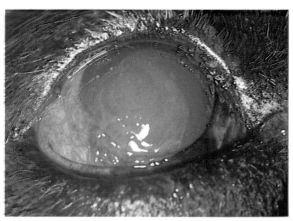

129

129 Corneal granulation tissue (Boxer, 7 years old) Following recurrent corneal erosion (*see also* **132** and **133**).

128 Corneal granulation tissue (Crossbred, 6 years old) Keratitis following a chemical burn.

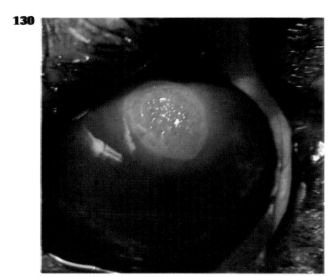

130

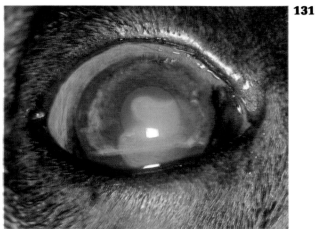

131

131 Corneal ulcer (Boxer, 8 years old) Stained with fluorescein to show the area of denuded epithelium.

130 Corneal granulation tissue (Chow, 8 months old) Associated with entropion. (See *also* **35.**)

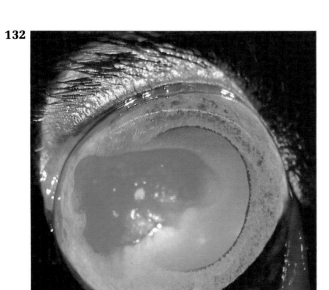

132 Corneal ulcer (Pembroke Corgi, 8 years old)
Stained with Rose Bengal to show devitalised
epithelium.

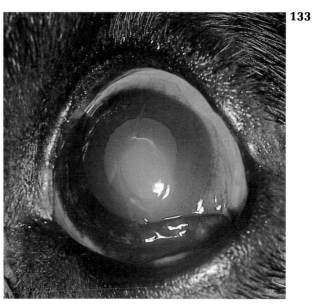

133 Corneal ulcer (Boxer, 7 years old) Recurrent
corneal erosion presenting as a painful and opaque
area.

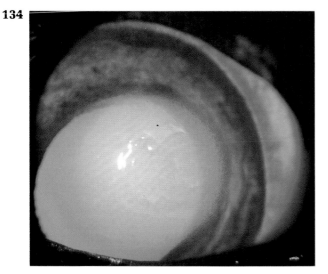

134 Corneal ulcer (Boxer, 8 years old) Recurrent
corneal erosion showing the edge of dead
epithelium.

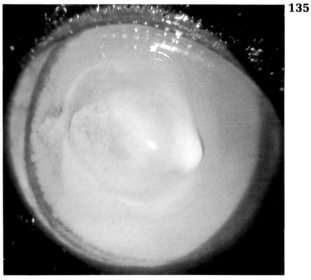

135 Corneal ulcer (Pug, 8 months old) Coagulase or
melting ulcer with oedema and vascular fringe.

136

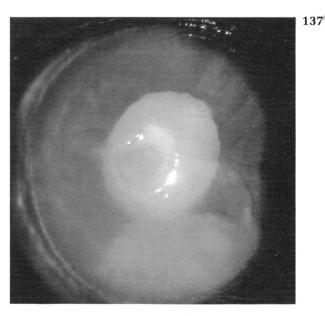

136 Corneal ulcer (Hunter, 7 years old) Coagulase ulcer. Note the gelatinous appearance of the corneal tissue.

137

137 Corneal ulcer (Pekingese, 6 years old) Deep ulcer and iritis (hypopyon and miosis).

138

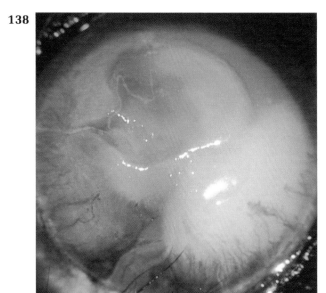

138 Corneal ulcer (Pekingese, 11 years old) Dense hypopyon and corneal vascularisation.

139

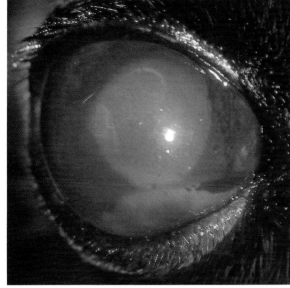

139 Corneal ulcer (Chihuahua, 8 years old) Hypopyon and hyphaema.

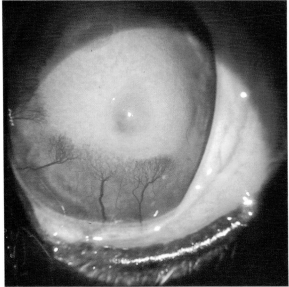

140 Corneal ulcer (Shih Tzu, 7 years old) A small keratocoele, corneal oedema and superficial vascularisation.

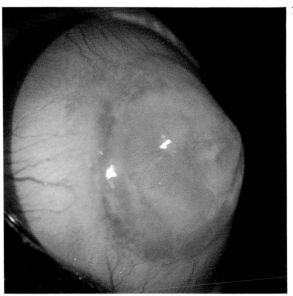

141 Corneal ulcer (Cavalier King Charles Spaniel, 4 years old) A large keratocoele and vascularisation.

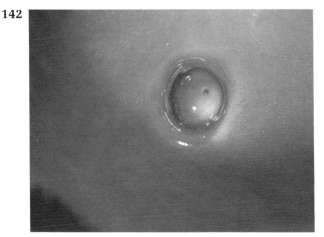

142 Corneal ulcer (Pekingese, 4 years old) A small, deep ulcer with clear keratocoele and early vascular fringe.

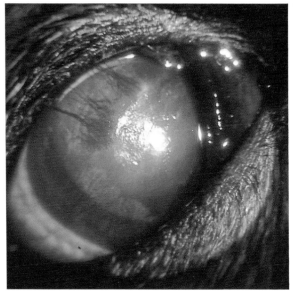

143 Corneal ulcer (Miniature Long-haired Dachshund, 8 years old) An ulcer secondary to facial paralysis.

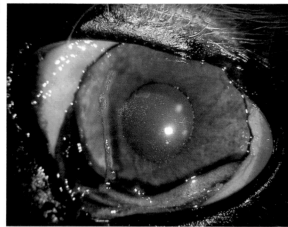

144 Keratoconjunctivitis sicca (West Highland White male, 3 years old) An early case with mucoid filaments on the cornea but no corneal pathology. Schirmer tear test zero.

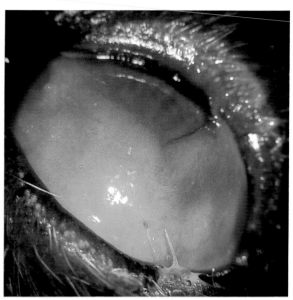

145 Keratoconjunctivitis sicca (West Highland White male, 8 years old) A moderately severe case with typical discharge.

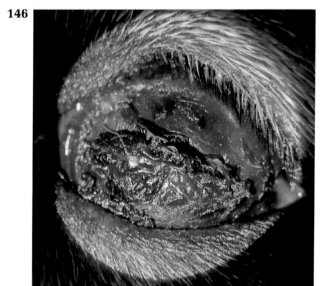

146 Keratoconjunctivitis sicca (Jack Russell Terrier female, 4 years old) A severe case.

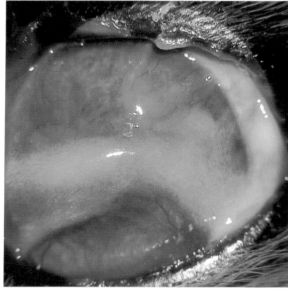

147 Keratoconjunctivitis sicca (Samoyed female, 6 years old) Typical discharge stuck on the cornea (compare with **98**).

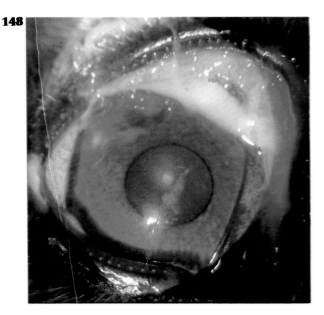

148 Keratoconjunctivitis sicca (West Highland White female, 2 years old) Discharge in the conjunctival fornix.

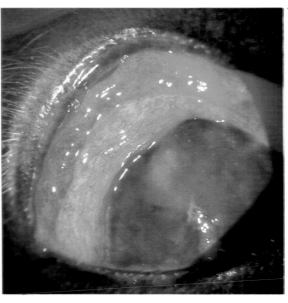

149 Keratoconjunctivitis sicca (Bichon Friese male, 3 years old) Conjunctival hyperplasia.

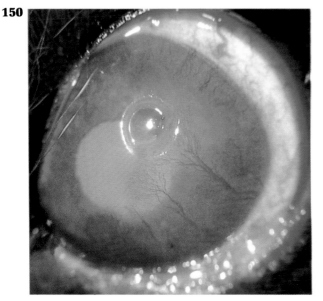

150 Keratoconjunctivitis sicca (West Highland White female, 7 years old) A typical deep circular ulcer and keratocoele.

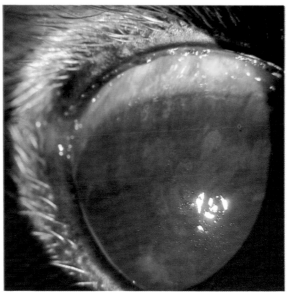

151 Keratoconjunctivitis sicca (West Highland White male, 5 years old) Secondary pigmentary keratitis.

152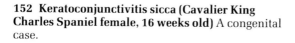

153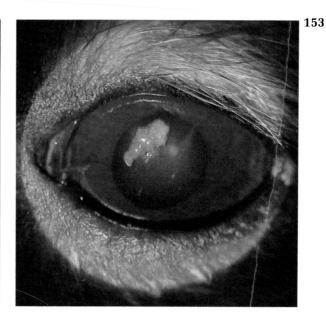

152 Keratoconjunctivitis sicca (Cavalier King Charles Spaniel female, 16 weeks old) A congenital case.

153 Keratoconjunctivitis sicca (Yorkshire Terrier female, 2 years old) An iatrogenic case following sulphasalazine therapy.

154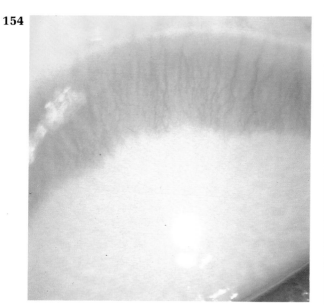

155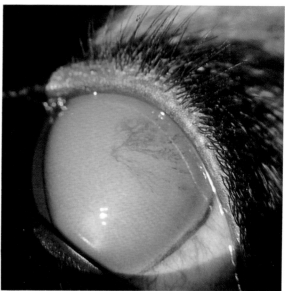

154 Corneal oedema (Airedale, 4 months old) Dense corneal oedema and vascular fringe, occurring 12 days after vaccination with live attenuated canine adenovirus-type 1 vaccine.

155 Corneal oedema (Long-haired Dachshund, 6 months old) Corneal oedema and corneal pigmentation. Another post-vaccination case.

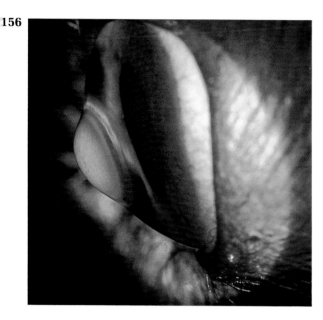

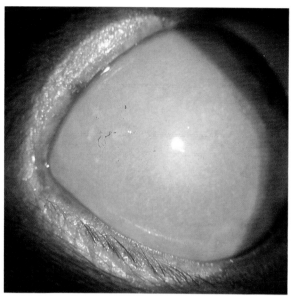

156 Corneal oedema (Yorkshire Terrier, 1 year old) Focal corneal oedema and associated keratoconus.

157 Corneal oedema (English Springer Spaniel, 9 years old) Corneal oedema and bullous keratopathy.

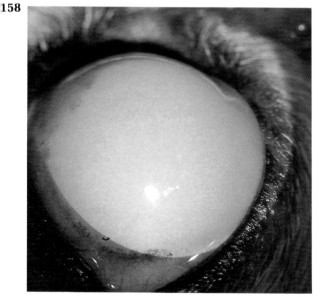

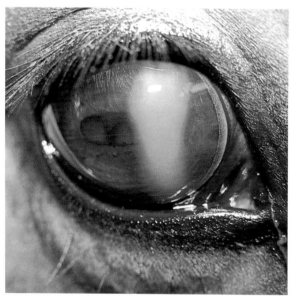

158 Corneal oedema (Chihuahua, 9 years old) Due to inherited corneal endothelial dystrophy.

159 Corneal oedema (Half-bred mare, 7 years old) Bilateral and asymmetrical partial oedema of unknown aetiology.

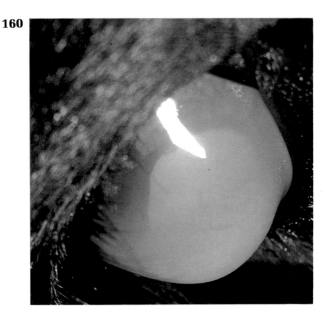

160 Corneal oedema (Friesian calf) Bilateral condition, hereditary in this breed. Again note keratoconus.

161 Corneal abscess (English Springer Spaniel, 3 years old)

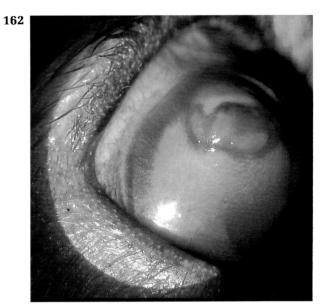

162 Corneal rupture (Cavalier King Charles Spaniel, 3 years old) Corneal rupture with iris prolapse, oedema and vascular fringe.

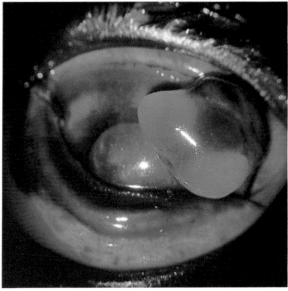

163 Corneal rupture (German Shepherd Dog, 10 weeks old) Corneal rupture plus coagulated aqueous following a cat scratch.

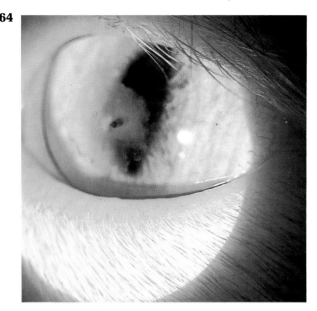

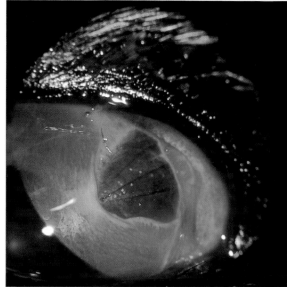

164 Corneal foreign body (DSH cat, 8 years old)
Note the cloud of leukocytes in the anterior chamber
around the foreign body.

**165 Corneal foreign body (Border Terrier, 7 years
old)** Leaf foreign body. Note the profound reaction
after 3 weeks.

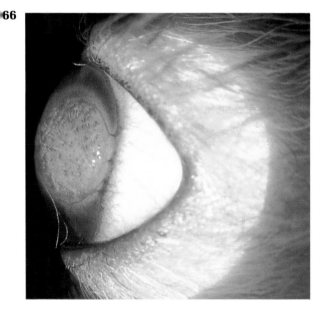

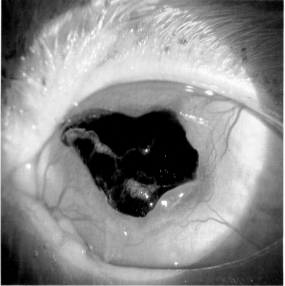

**166 Corneal dermoid (German Shepherd Dog, 3
months old)** See also **16-18**.

**167 Corneal sequestrum (Colourpoint cat, 2 years
old)** Bilateral case. Note large sequestrum together
with corneal vascularisation and granulation tissue
lifting the edge of the sequestrum.

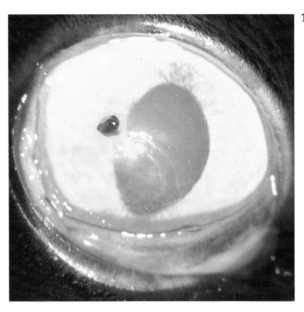

168 Corneal sequestrum (Colourpoint cat, 13 months old) Medium-size sequestrum and no vascularisation.

169 Corneal sequestrum (Burmese cat, 9 years old) Very small raised sequestrum.

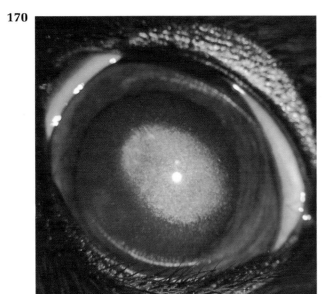

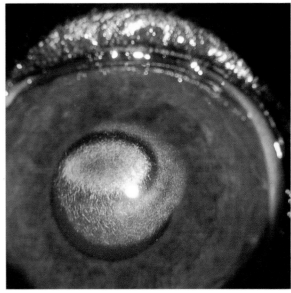

170 Lipid keratopathy (Rough Collie male, 3 years old) Bilateral, approximately symmetrical, corneal lipidosis.

171 Lipid keratopathy (Cavalier King Charles Spaniel female, 3 years old) Corneal lipidosis. Typical age, breed and sex.

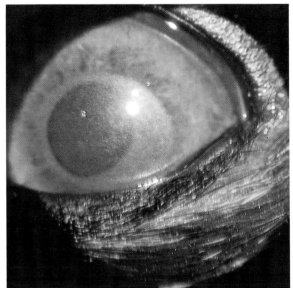

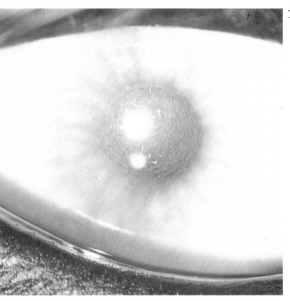

172 Lipid keratopathy (Cavalier King Charles Spaniel female, 3 years old) Corneal lipidosis, larger and less dense than that shown in the previous figure.

173 Lipid keratopathy (Siberian Husky female, 3 years old) Corneal dystrophy.

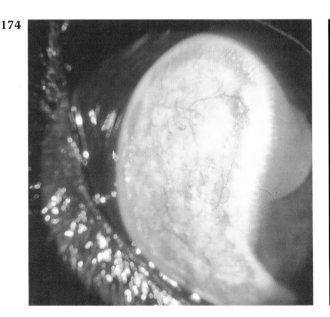

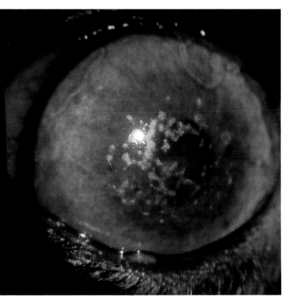

174 Lipid keratopathy (Golden Retriever female, 3 years old) Corneal degeneration. A perilimbal calcified lesion with epithelial involvement and vascularisation.

175 Lipid keratopathy (Miniature Wire-haired Dachshund female, 2 years old) Associated with distichiasis.

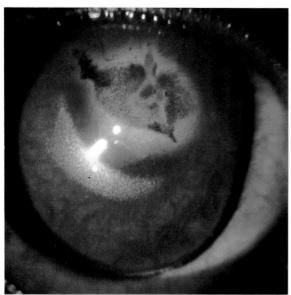

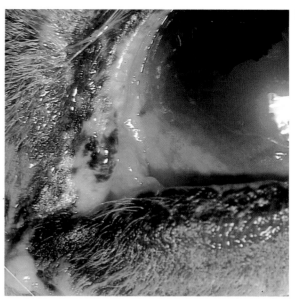

176 Lipid keratopathy (Pug, 13 months old)
Associated with corneal scar, pigment and anterior synechiae.

177 Corneal tumour—squamous cell carcinoma (Hunter, 10 years old)

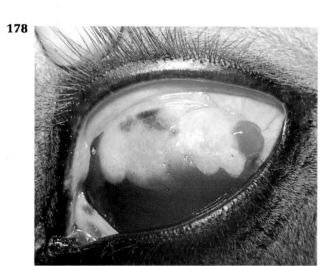

178 Corneal tumour—squamous cell carcinoma (pony, 9 years old)

The Iris

Iritis, or anterior uveitis, is an important and painful eye condition, often difficult to diagnose and of an obscure aetiology. In this section the clinical signs of iritis, of varying causes in the dog, cat and horse, are illustrated. In the dog the association with cataract, vascularisation, haemorrhage and synechiae are shown. In the cat iritis is not uncommon and can be due to toxoplasmosis, feline infectious peritonitis and multicentric lymphosarcoma. In the horse iritis, as equine periodic ophthalmia or recurrent uveitis, is most important in relation to purchase and soundness.

This section also records congenital conditions such as colobomata and persistent pupillary membranes in both the dog and horse. In these same species and in the cat uveal cysts are illustrated, and in the horse the similarity with hyperplasia of the corpora nigra can be compared.

Intraocular tumours commonly affect the uveal tract in the domestic species and various examples of iris and ciliary body tumours are also included.

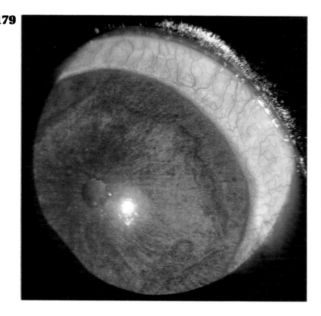

179 Iritis (Cavalier King Charles Spaniel, 10 years old) Acute iritis (traumatic). Note marked miosis and conjunctival injection.

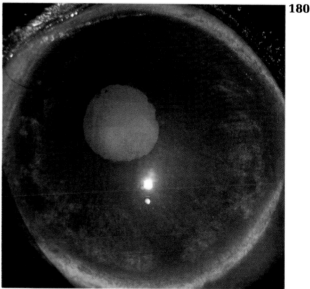

180 Iritis (Miniature Poodle, 10 years old) Chronic iritis. Note dark iris, miosis, cataract and pigment on anterior lens capsule.

181

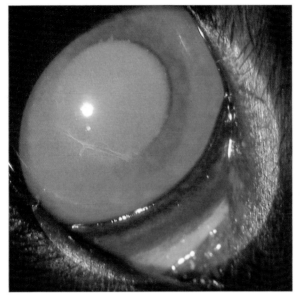

181 Iritis (Airedale, 2 years old) Acute iritis showing plastic endothelial deposit and flare.

182

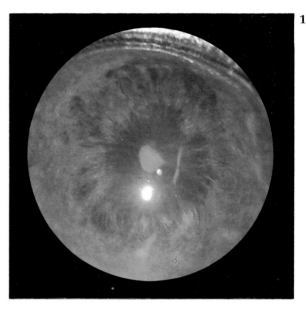

182 Iritis (Crossbred, 4 years old) Traumatic iritis. Note swollen iris, miosis and haemorrhage.

183

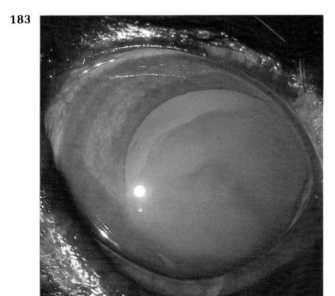

183 Iritis (Crossbred, 14 years old) Note haemorrhage and dull iris.

184

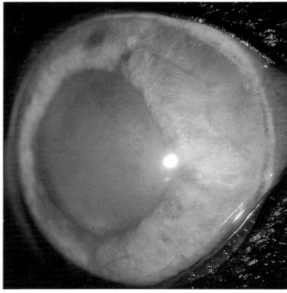

184 Iritis (Border Collie, 9 years old) Iris bombé due to posterior synechiae and secondary glaucoma.

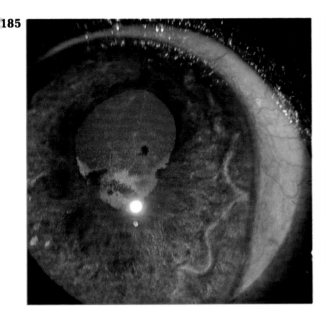

185 Iritis (Cavalier King Charles, 4 years old)
Posterior synechiae and eccentric pupil.

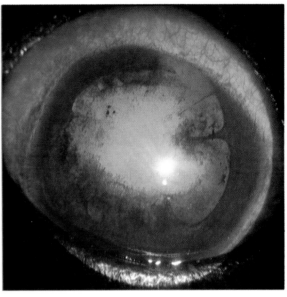

186 Iritis (Miniature Poodle, 10 years old) Posterior synechiae and cataract (pupil dilated with 1% Tropicamide).

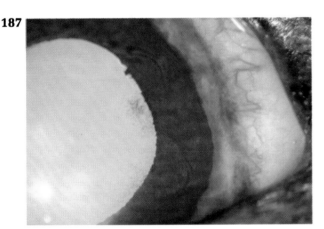

187 Iritis (Jack Russell Terrier, 6 years old)
Posterior synechiae following uveitis and secondary glaucoma.

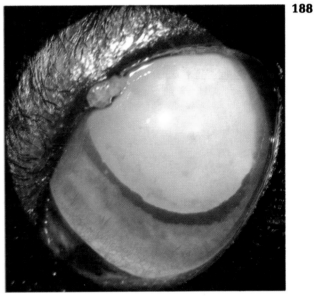

188 Iritis (Miniature Poodle, 6 years old) Cataract and haemorrhage on lens, vascular corneal fringe and herniated uveal pigment around pupil edge.

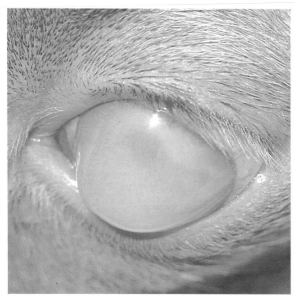

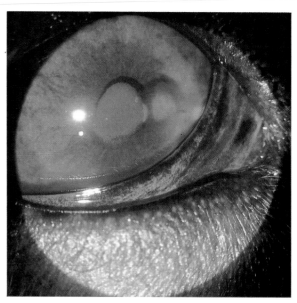

189 Iritis (Weimaraner, 3 months old) Note miosis, corneal oedema and keratoconus (*see also* **156**).

190 Iritis (Labrador cross, 3 years old) Penetrating corneal injury. Note the foreign body, flare, miosis and herniation of the posterior uveal pigment.

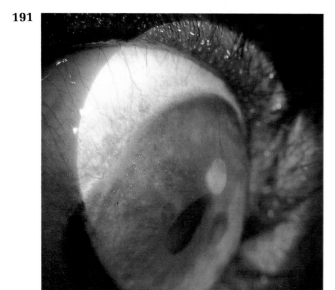

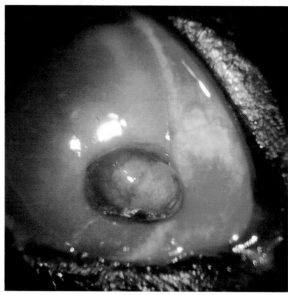

191 Iritis (Pekingese, 2 years old) Penetrating corneal injury with anterior synechia and corneal scar.

192 Iritis (English Springer Spaniel, 3 years old) Iris prolapse following a shot injury.

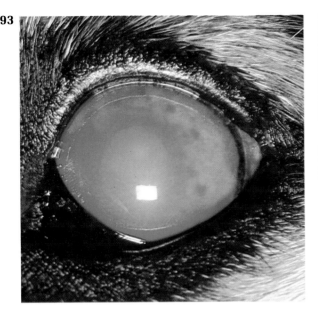

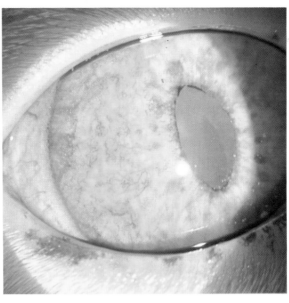

193 Iritis (German Shepherd Dog, 3 years old)
Ehrlichiosis. Note the multiple haemorrhages on the
iris and corneal oedema.

194 Iritis (DSH cat, 15 years old) Note the
congested blood vessels on the iris.

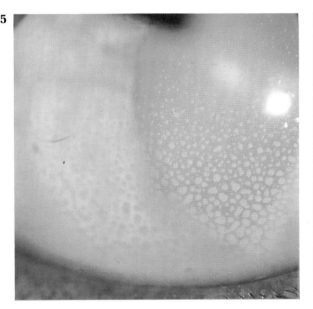

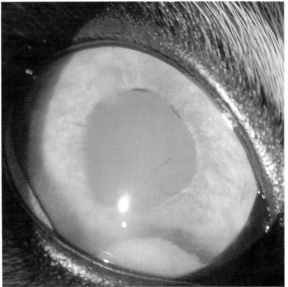

195 Iritis (DSH cat, 15 years old) Note keratitis
precipitata (KP). A toxoplasma case.

196 Iritis (DSH cat, 10 years old) Note hypopyon
and blood vessels on the anterior lens capsule. The
aetiology was unknown but associated with some
systemic illness.

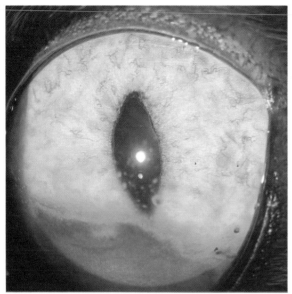

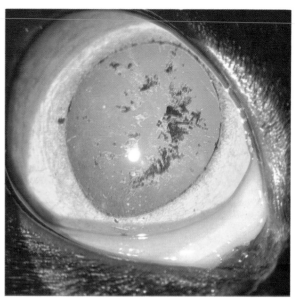

197 Iritis (DSH cat, 8 years old) Note hyphaema and vascular engorgement of the iris. A toxoplasma case.

198 Iritis (DSH cat, 18 months old) Note the posterior synechiae.

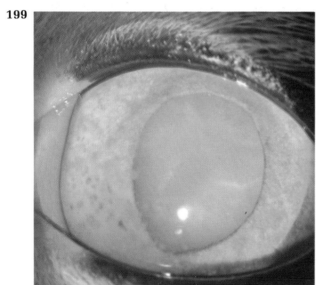

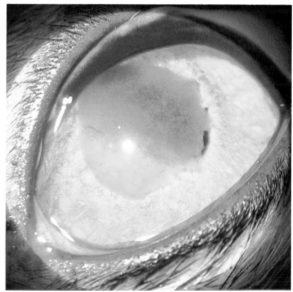

199 Iritis (DSH cat, 5 years old) Note cataract and KP. Feline infectious peritonitis case.

200 Iritis (DSH cat, 10 months old) Note hypopyon, miosis, posterior synechiae and irregular pupil. A toxoplasma case.

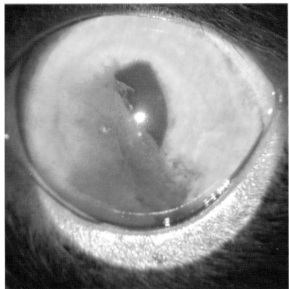

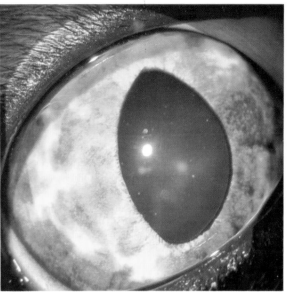

201 Iritis (DSH cat, 1 year old) Note hyphaema.
Feline infectious peritonitis case.

202 Iris freckles (DSH cat, 6 years old) Progressive
loss of anterior iris pigment with resulting darker
spots. Unknown aetiology.

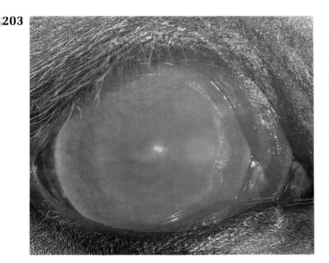

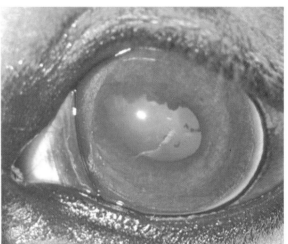

**203 Iritis—equine periodic ophthalmia
(Connemara pony, 3 years old)** Dull and faintly
opaque cornea and miosis.

**204 Iritis—equine periodic ophthalmia
(Thoroughbred, 3 years old)** Irregular pupil due to
posterior synechiae.

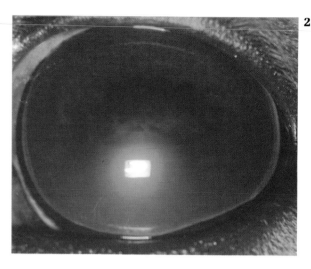

**206 Iritis—equine periodic ophthalmia
(Thoroughbred, 6 years old)** Occlusion of the pupil.

**205 Iritis—equine periodic ophthalmia
(Thoroughbred, 12 years old)** Posterior synechiae
and cataract.

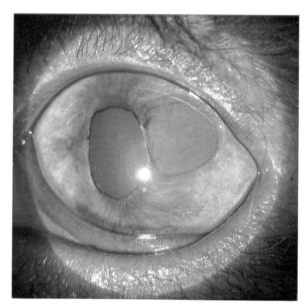

207 Iris coloboma (Miniature Poodle, 5 years old)
Mid-iris complete coloboma at 10 o'clock. The
cataract is unrelated.

208 Iris coloboma (Miniature Poodle, 3 years old)
Partial coloboma at 2 o'clock. Note the distortion of
the pupil shape.

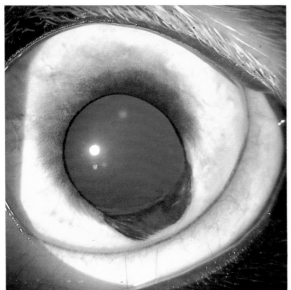

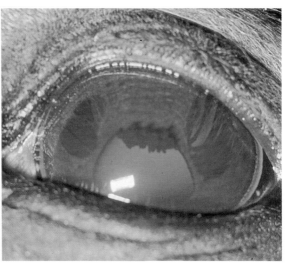

210 Iris coloboma (Pony, 5 years old) Complete (1 o'clock) and partial (10 o'clock) colobomata. Both eyes of this animal were affected, but asymmetrically.

209 Iris coloboma (Great Dane, 3 months old, blue merle) Partial coloboma at the typical position of 6 o'clock; pale blue iris. Note the red fundus reflex.

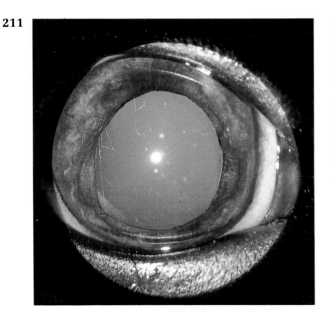

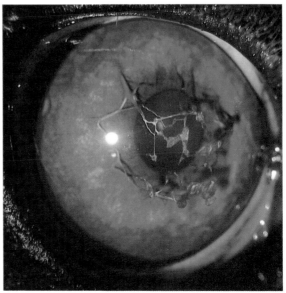

211 Iris—congenital anomalies (Rottweiler, 11 weeks old) Irregular pupil due to iris hypoplasia and pupillary membranes.

212 Persistent pupillary membranes (Labrador, 6 months old) Multiple persistent pupillary membranes, or congenital anterior synechiae, with focal corneal opacities.

213

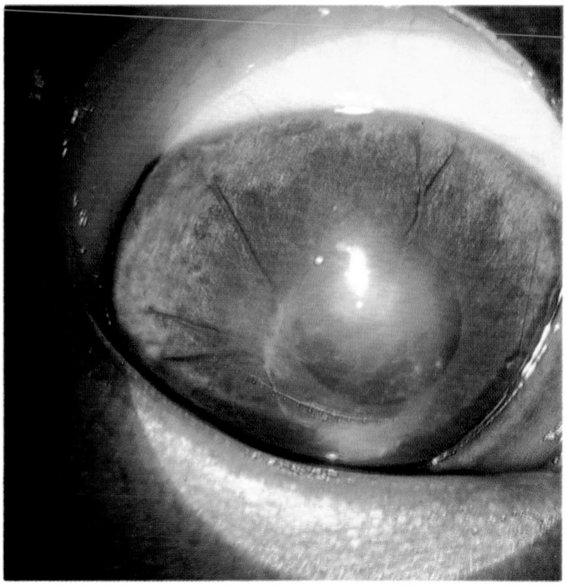

213 Persistent pupillary membranes (Beagle, 3 months old) Similar to the previous figure but less severe and with a diffuse corneal opacity.

214

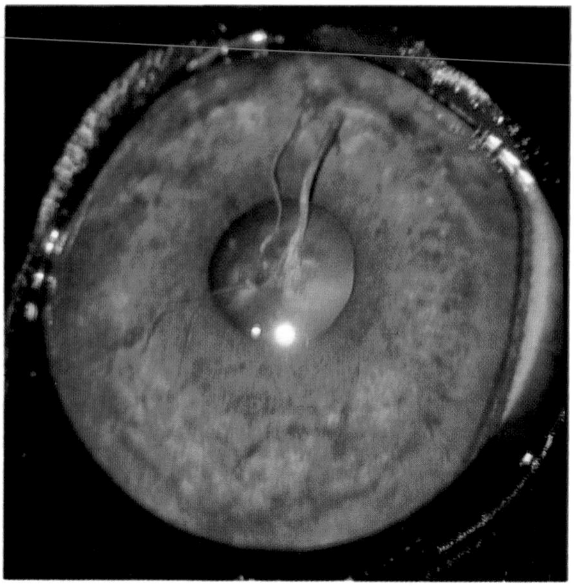

214 Persistent pupillary membranes (Cairn Terrier, 6 years old) Persistent pupillary membranes to anterior lens capsule with associated focal cataracts.

215

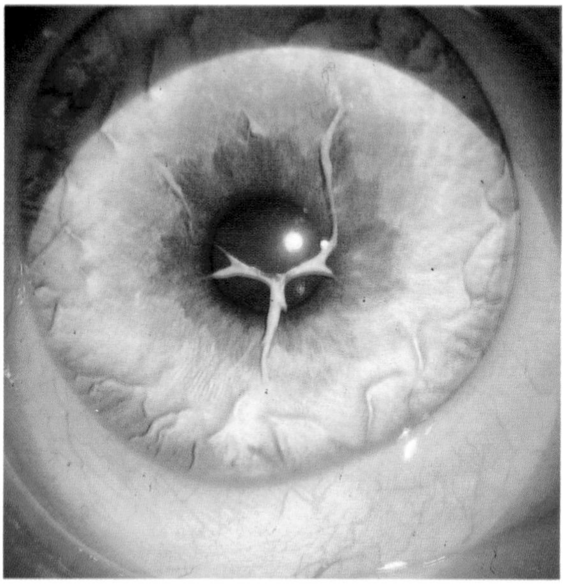

215 Persistent pupillary membranes (Old English Sheepdog, 3 months old) Persistent pupillary membranes in a pale blue iris.

216

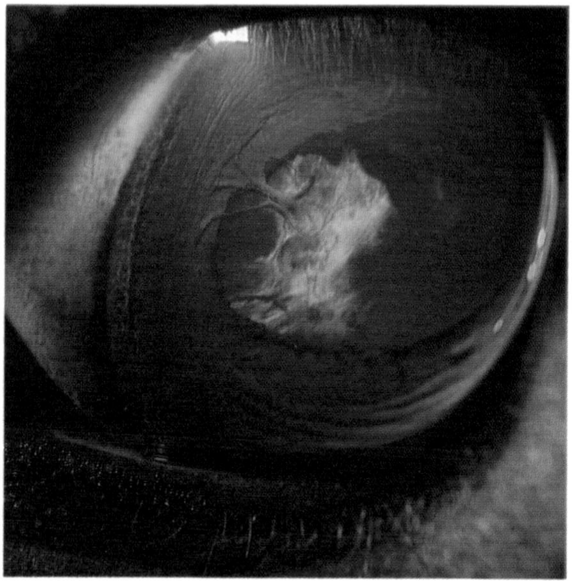

216 Persistent pupillary membranes (Part Arab mare, 8 years old) Persistent pupillary membranes and associated pigmented capsular cataract.

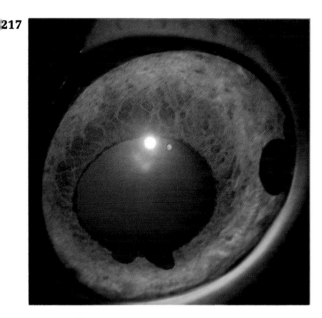

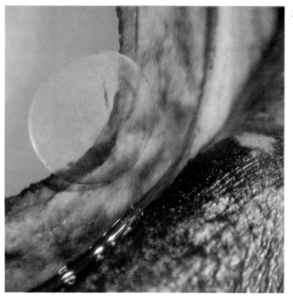

217 Uveal cysts (Crossbred, 7 years old) A few dense cysts both free and attached.

218 Uveal cyst (Labrador, 4 years old) A single thin-walled cyst.

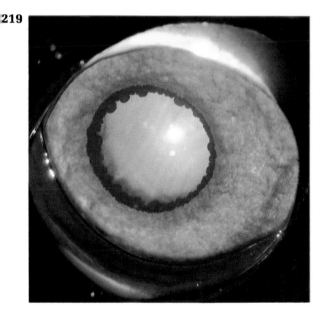

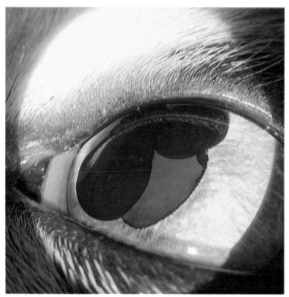

219 Uveal cysts (Labrador, 9 months old) Cataract and associated cysts around the pupillary border following iritis.

220 Uveal cysts (DSH cat, 5 years old) Free cysts in the anterior chamber.

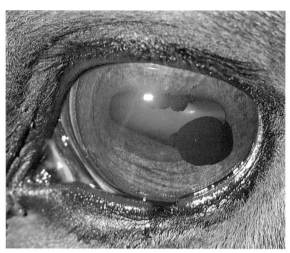

221 Uveal cysts (Hunter, 9 years old) Attached to the pupillary margin.

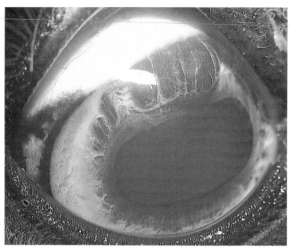

222 Uveal cysts (Welsh pony, grey, 7 years old) Cystic mass in the superior mid-iris region in blue iris.

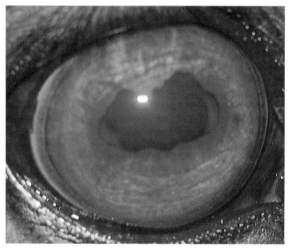

223 Corpora nigra hyperplasia (Hunter gelding, 13 years old) Note the complete obliteration of the centre part of the pupil. The other eye showed no abnormality.

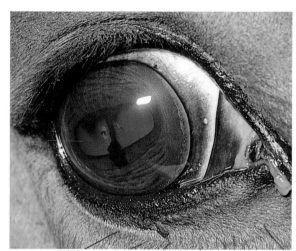

224 Corpora nigra trauma (Thoroughbred, 4 years old) 'Whiplash'-type injury resulting in tearing of the corpora nigra.

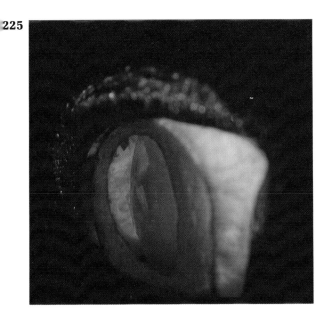

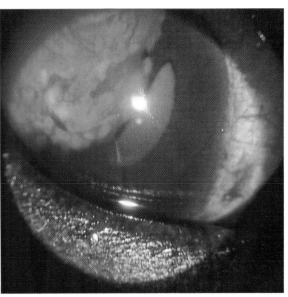

225 Ciliary body tumour—adenoma (Labrador, 9 years old) Note the small haemorrhage on the anterior lens capsule.

226 Ciliary body tumour—adenocarcinoma (Staffordshire Bull Terrier, 6 years old) Unpigmented pink mass in the anterior chamber, with distortion of the pupil.

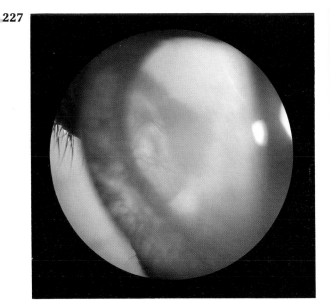

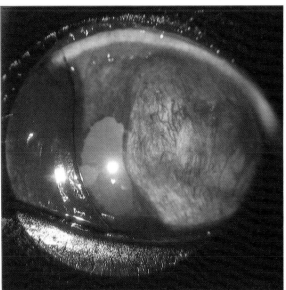

227 Ciliary body tumour—adenocarcinoma (Greyhound, 7 years old) The appearance of the tumour through the pupil.

228 Ciliary body tumour—melanoma (Afghan, 7 years old) Large swelling with distortion of the pupil.

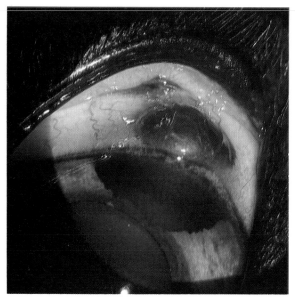

229 Ciliary body tumour—malignant melanoma (Labrador, 2 years old) Involvement of the iris, ciliary body and choroid.

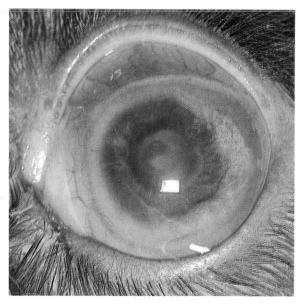

230 Iris tumour—multicentric lymphosarcoma (English Springer Spaniel, 5 years old) Causing secondary glaucoma due to obliteration of the angle of filtration.

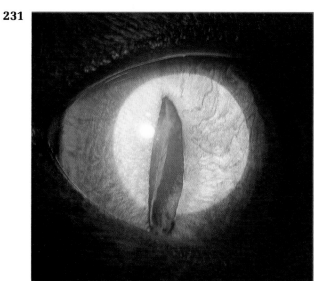

231 Iris tumour—melanoma (DSH cat, 7 years old) Pigmented mass appearing in the pupil. Note also the increased vascularisation of the iris on that side.

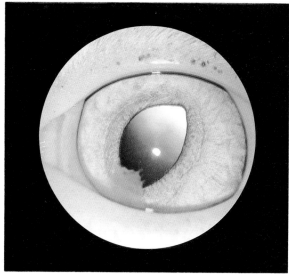

232 Iris tumour—multicentric lymphosarcoma (DSH cat, 2 years old) Neoplastic cells in the anterior chamber. The other eye was more severely affected.

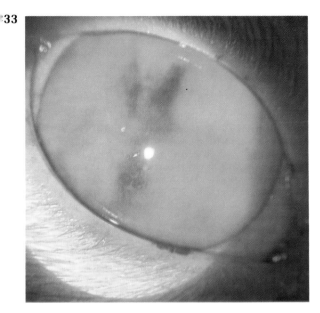

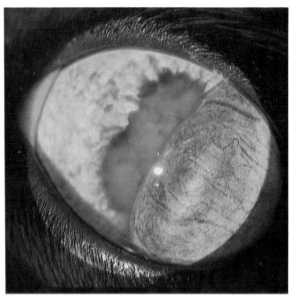

**233 Iris tumour—multicentric lymphosarcoma
(DSH cat, 16 years old)** Also kidney involvement.

**234 Iris tumour—multicentric lymphosarcoma
(DSH cat, 3 years old)**

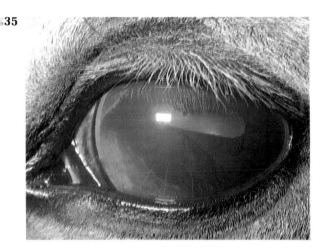

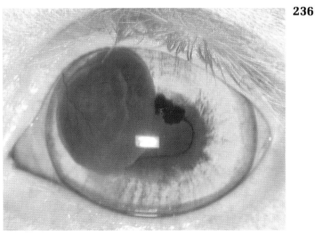

**235 Iris tumour—melanoma (Grey pony, 13 years
old)**

**236 Iris tumour—amelanotic melanoma (Blue-eyed
cream pony, 7 years old)**

Glaucoma

Glaucoma (increased intraocular pressure) is another important and painful eye condition and, without subjective symptoms and tonometry and gonioscopy, it is difficult to diagnose in animals. The clinical signs of glaucoma are shown in the following series of slides; the breed and age of each case should be carefully noted, as this information may well suggest a diagnosis of primary (hereditary) glaucoma (see **237** to **244**). Examples of goniophotographs of the normal (open) angle and its variations are compared with the appearance of the closed angle in primary glaucoma in the Welsh Springer Spaniel.

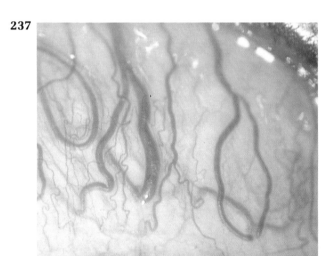

237 Conjunctival congestion (Beagle female, 9 years old)

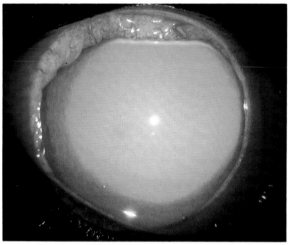

238 Conjunctival chemosis (Welsh Springer Spaniel female, 18 months old)

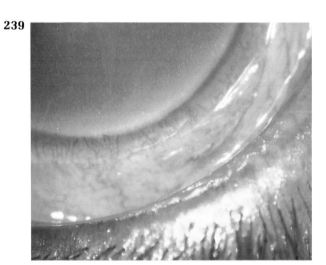

239 Early vascular fringe (English Springer Spaniel male, 11 years old)

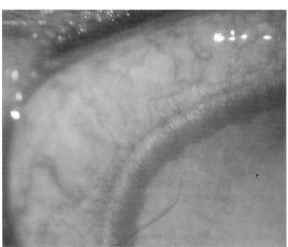

240 Later vascular fringe (Welsh Springer Spaniel female, 9 months old)

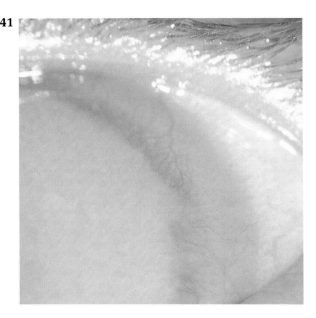

241 Late fringe and corneal oedema (Miniature Poodle female, 11 years old)

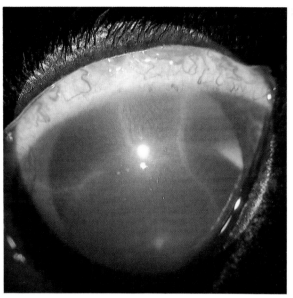

242 Fractures in Descemet's membrane (Basset Hound female, 7 years old)

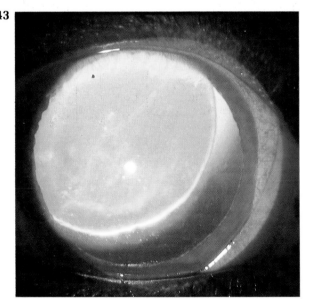

243 Secondary dislocation of the lens (Welsh Springer Spaniel female, 4 years old) Primary glaucoma with secondary lens dislocation—note the direction of this lens dislocation. Compare with **340** and **341**.

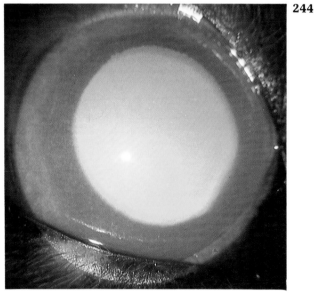

244 Dilated pupil and "steamy" cornea (Welsh Springer Spaniel female, 5 years old)

245

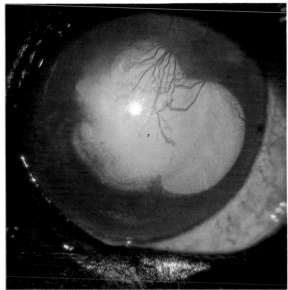

246

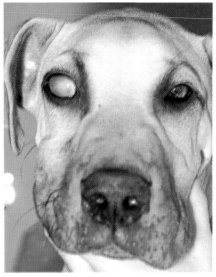

245 Posterior synechiae (Standard Schnauzer female, 14 years old) Post-iritis glaucoma with adhesions resulting in eccentric and dilated pupil.

246 Hydrophthalmos or absolute glaucoma (Great Dane, 7 months old) Uveitis associated with CAV-1 vaccination and secondary glaucoma (*see* **10, 154** and **155**).

247

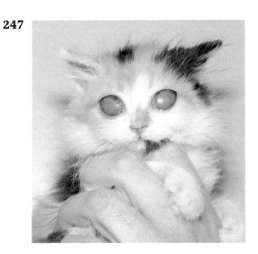

248

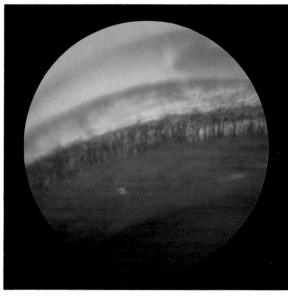

247 Buphthalmos or congenital glaucoma (DSH cat female, 9 weeks old)

248 Goniophotograph—open angle (Irish Setter female, 1 year old)

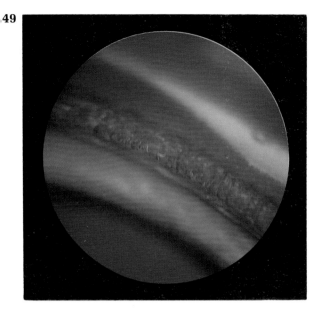

249 Goniophotograph—open angle (Crossbred female, 3 years old)

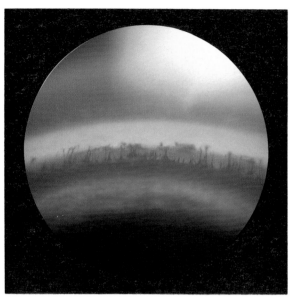

250 Goniophotograph—open angle (Welsh Springer Spaniel female, 6 years old)

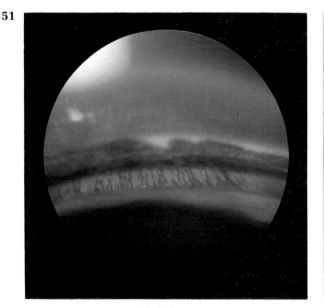

251 Goniophotograph—open angle (Welsh Springer Spaniel male, 2 years old)

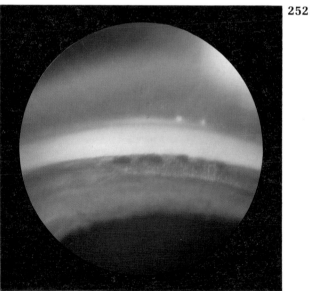

252 Goniophotograph—closed angle (Welsh Springer Spaniel female, 4 years old)

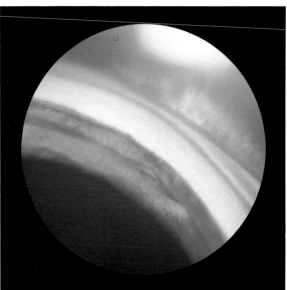

253 Goniophotograph—closed angle (Welsh Springer Spaniel female, 4 years old)

254 Goniophotograph—closed angle (Welsh Springer Spaniel male, 4 years old)

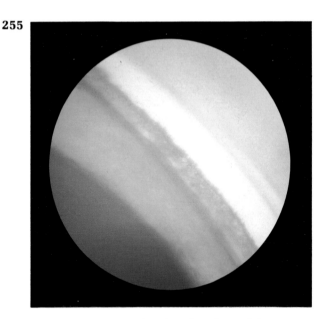

255 Goniophotograph—closed angle (Welsh Springer Spaniel female, 2 years old)

The Lens

The two main conditions affecting the lens, cataract and luxation, are dealt with separately.

Cataracts

Cataracts are divided into a number of categories. The first, and largest, category covers primary, hereditary, non-congenital cataracts *i.e.* cataracts which are not present at birth but which develop later in life, are not associated with any other eye disease and are inherited. In this group the breed incidence is of particular importance and several examples are given, demonstrating the progression of the cataract and its appearance at different ages in the breeds mainly affected.

The second group of cataracts are congenital (present at birth) and are usually, if not invariably, associated with some other ocular anomaly, particularly microphthalmos. Some of these cataracts have been proven to be inherited (Miniature Schnauzer), whilst others are suspected of being inherited as they show a strong breed predisposition (Cavalier King Charles Spaniel and English Cocker Spaniel). Others would seem to be isolated examples of a congenital non-inherited anomaly (crossbred).

The third group includes cataracts secondary to systemic disease, such as diabetes, and to nutritional and toxic effects. A further category includes those occurring secondary to other ocular disease, such as generalised and central progressive retinal atrophy, retinal dysplasia and glaucoma. Traumatic cataracts are also included in this group, as well as resorbing cataracts associated with uveitis and cataracts occurring in conjunction with non-hereditary ocular anomalies such as lenticonus, coloboma and hyaloid artery. Finally, three unusual forms of cataract are illustrated.

The last group deals with false cataracts - lens opacities which on examination, can easily be confused with true cataracts.

Lens Luxation

Lens luxation is illustrated by the clinical signs of vitreous in the pupil, the aphakic crescent and the gross appearance of anterior and posterior dislocation. Obviously iridodonesis cannot be shown. The appearance of glaucoma secondary to lens luxation is also illustrated. Three cases of lens luxation in the cat are included.

Primary Hereditary Non-Congenital Cataracts

256 Golden Retriever (1 year old) Posterior polar, subcapsular, dense focal opacity.

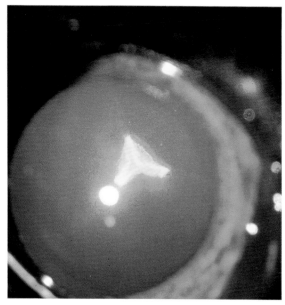

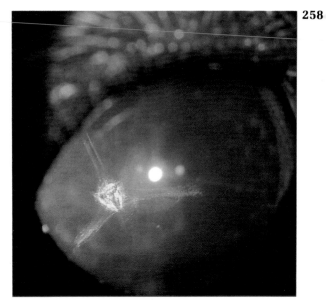

257 Golden Retriever (4 years old) Posterior polar, subcapsular, faint inverted-Y opacity.

258 Golden Retriever (18 months old) Posterior polar, subcapsular, dense triangle with extensions along suture lines.

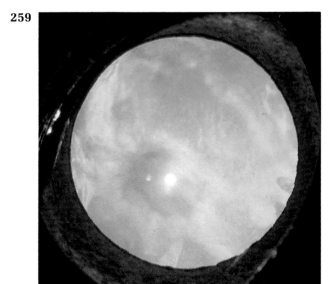

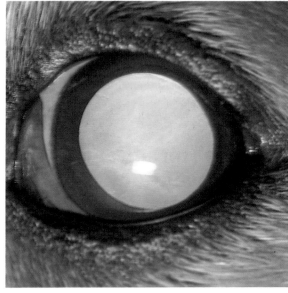

259 Golden Retriever (4 years old) Cortical opacities and dense posterior polar cataract.

260 Golden Retriever (2 years old) Total cataract.

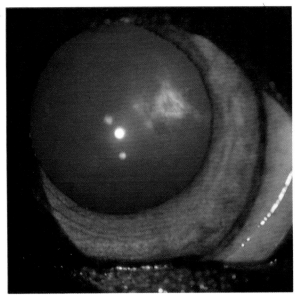

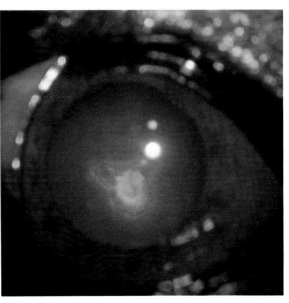

261 Labrador Retriever (3 years old) Posterior polar subcapsular cataract.

262 Labrador Retriever (6 years old) Dam of the animal shown in the previous figure.

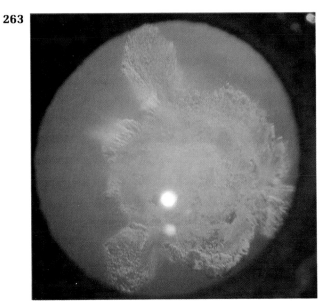

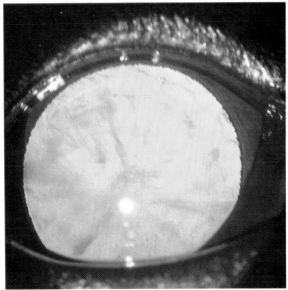

263 Labrador Retriever (9 years old) Large posterior polar cataract with extensions.

264 Labrador Retriever (4 years old) Total cataract. Note the density of inverted-Y suture lines.

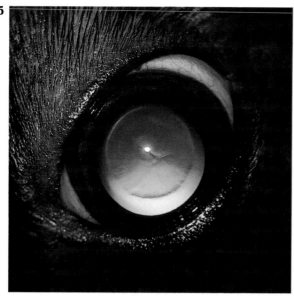

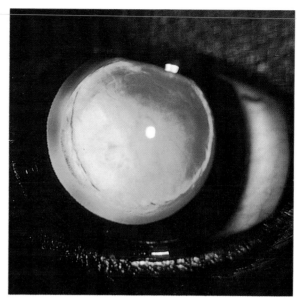

265 Boston Terrier (8 weeks old) Central opacity, bilaterally symmetrical.

266 Boston Terrier (4 months old) Progression of central bilaterally symmetrical opacity.

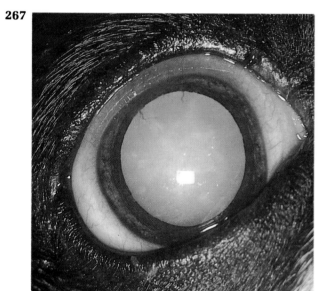

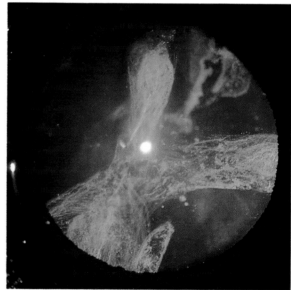

267 Boston Terrier (3 years old) Total mature cataract.

268 Boston Terrier (6 years old) Late-onset type cataract.

269

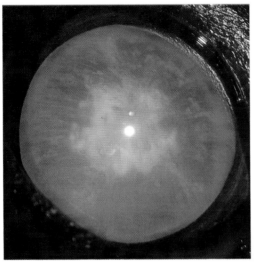

270

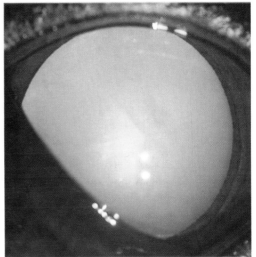

271

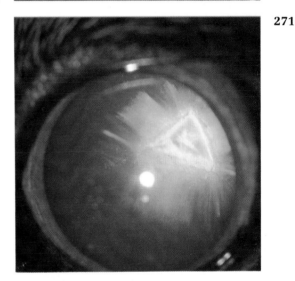

269 Staffordshire Bull Terrier (2 years old)
Bilateral symmetrical progressive cataract, very
similar in appearance to the first type in the Boston
Terrier (**265-267**)

270 Afghan Hound (2 years old) Bilateral cataracts,
symmetrical and total.

271 Norwegian Buhund (10 months old) Posterior
polar cataract with extension.

272 Norwegian Buhund (6 months old) Large
posterior polar opacity.

273 Norwegian Buhund (21 months old)
Progressive, peripheral cortical cataract plus
posterior polar cataract.

272

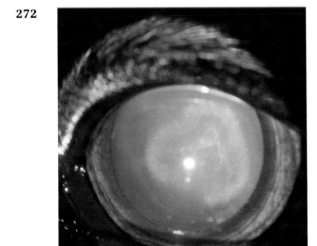

273

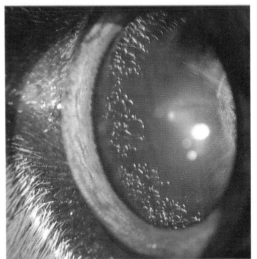

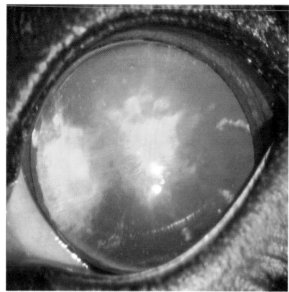

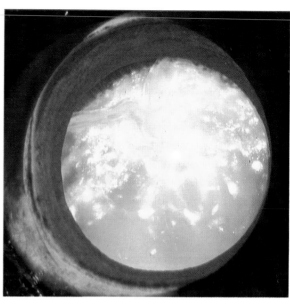

274 American Cocker Spaniel (3 years old) Focal cataracts. Cataract in this breed is often asymmetrical.

275 American Cocker Spaniel (5 years old) Lens resorbtion with folding of the capsule.

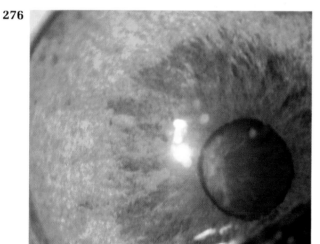

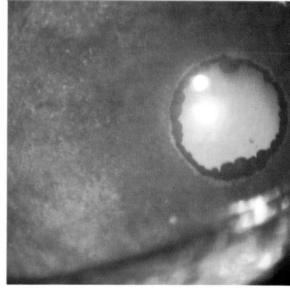

276 American Cocker Spaniel (3 years old) Partial cataract. Note the normal iris colour.

277 American Cocker Spaniel (4 years old) Total cataract with associated uveitis. Note iris colour and pupillary cysts.

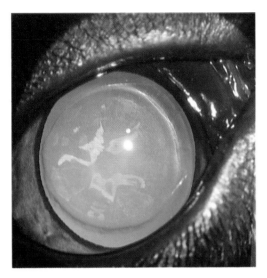

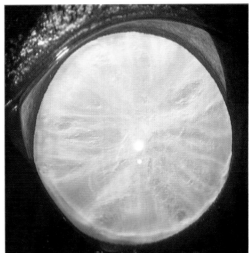

278 German Shepherd Dog (4 months old) This cataract is progressive.

279 German Shepherd Dog (9 months old) The two eyes are not always identical.

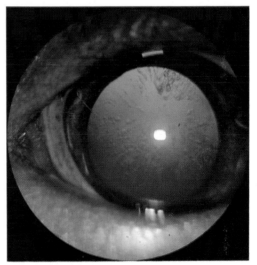

280 Welsh Springer Spaniel (8 weeks old) Bilateral, symmetrical and progressive cataract.

281 Standard Poodle (12 months old) Bilateral and progressive; the two eyes are similar.

282 Cavalier King Charles Spaniel (18 months old) Bilateral, total and progressive cataract. Not congenital (*see also* **286-289**).

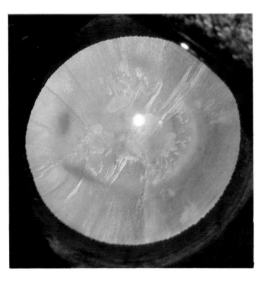

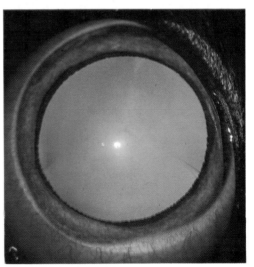

Congenital Cataract and Associated Anomalies

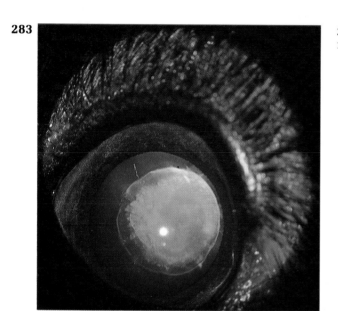

283 Miniature Schnauzer (6 months old) Bilateral microphthalmos and nuclear cataract.

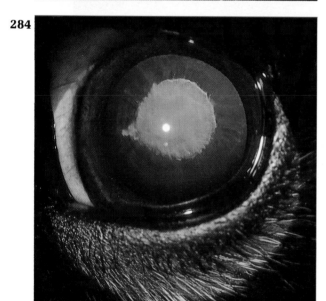

284 Miniature Schnauzer (6 months old) Nuclear cataract with extension.

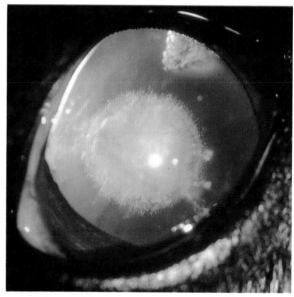

285 Miniature Schnauzer (14 months old) Nuclear cataract plus cortical wedge.

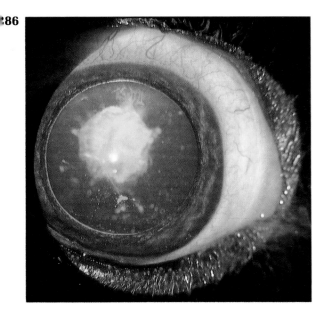

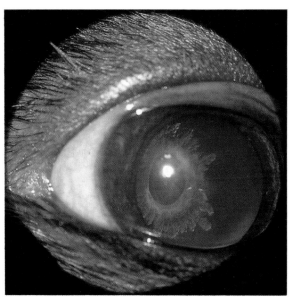

286 Cavalier King Charles Spaniel (6 months old)
Microphthalmos plus nuclear and anterior capsular cataract.

287 Cavalier King Charles Spaniel (7 weeks old)
Cataract and posterior lenticonus.

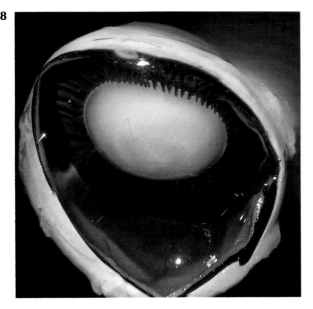

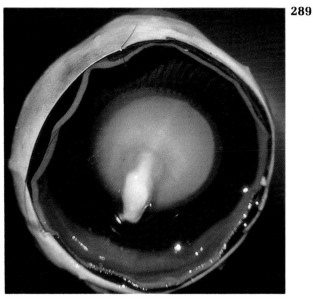

288 Cavalier King Charles Spaniel (7 weeks old)
Post-mortem specimen showing mild posterior lenticonus. The same eye as shown in the previous figure.

289 Cavalier King Charles Spaniel (7 weeks old)
Marked posterior lentiglobus. The other eye of the same dog as shown in the previous figure.

290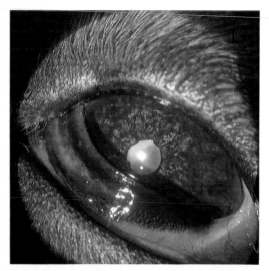

290 Cocker Spaniel (14 weeks old) Cataract, microphthalmos and prominence of the nictitating membrane, together with iris hypoplasia.

291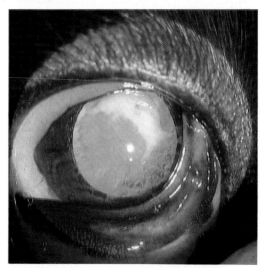

291 Cocker Spaniel (14 weeks old) Litter mate to the animal shown in the previous figure showing the extent of the cataract following mydriasis.

292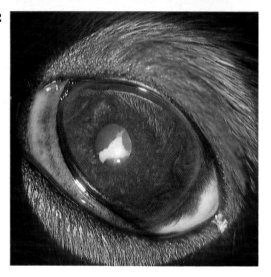

292 Cocker Spaniel (10 weeks old) Microphthalmos and dense, white, anterior capsular, sometimes pyramidal, cataract.

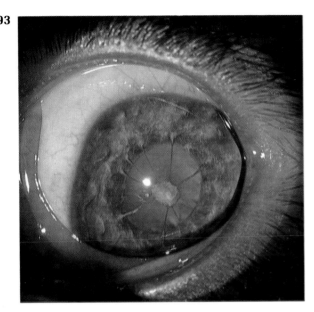

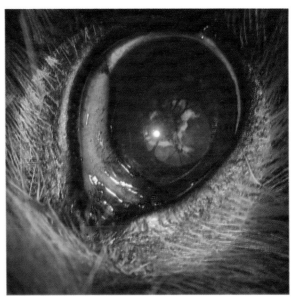

293 English Springer Spaniel (13 weeks old)
Microphthalmos, congenital cataract and persistent pupillary membranes.

294 West Highland White (11 weeks old)
Microphthalmos, congenital cataract and persistent pupillary membranes.

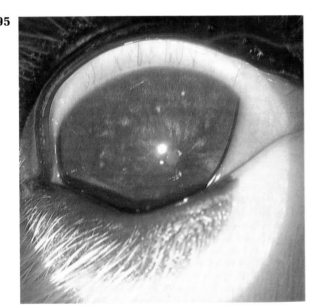

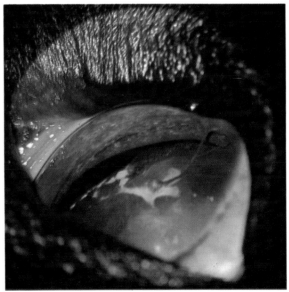

295 Old English Sheepdog (9 months old)
Microphthalmos and cataract. Note the marked miosis and uveal cysts.

296 Crossbred (11 months old) Microphthalmos, cataract, persistent pupillary membranes, lens coloboma and poor limbal differentiation.

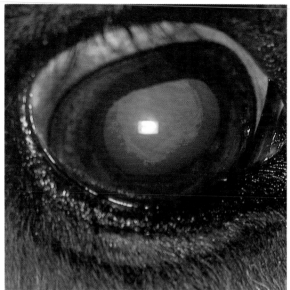 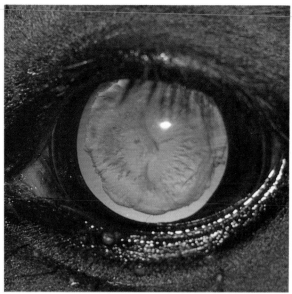

297 Nuclear cataract (Friesian calf) Congenital and bilateral.

298 Congenital cataract (Arab foal) Congenital cataract in the Arabian horse is much more common than in the Thoroughbred. In this animal the cataract is nuclear but it may take other forms.

Other Types of Cataract

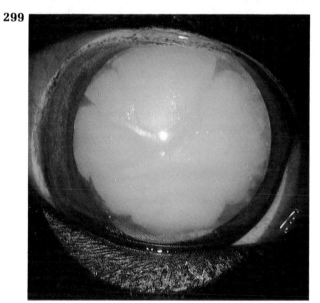 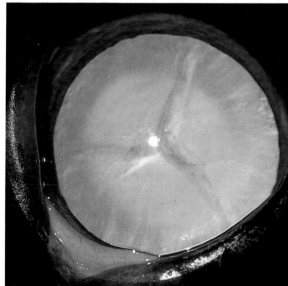

299 Diabetic cataract (Crossbred, 12 years old) Bilateral, symmetrical and frequently sudden in onset. Note the water clefts.

300 Diabetic cataract (Pembroke Corgi, 9 years old) Presenile type—slower in onset than previous type.

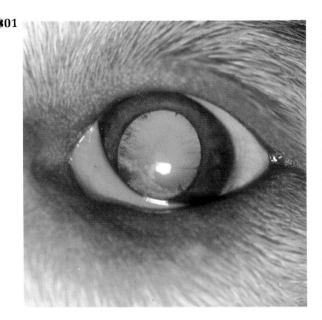

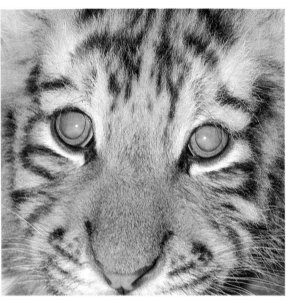

301 Nutritional cataract (Foxhound puppy)
Probably due to a deficiency of the vitamin B
complex. Congenital.

302 Nutritional cataract (Tiger cub) Bilateral
cataract in a hand-reared animal.

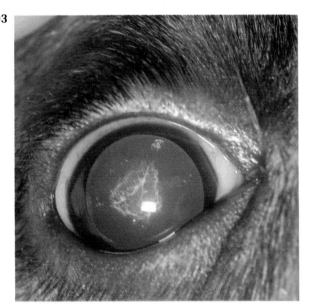

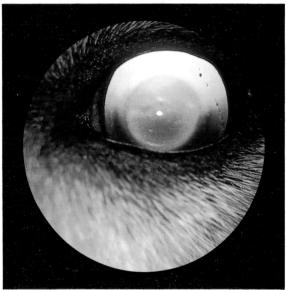

303 Toxic cataract (Beagle, young adult) Cataract is
a common finding in toxicity trials and can be
caused by many compounds.

304 Toxic cataract (Beagle, young adult) Unusual
appearance of the lens due to dimethyl sulphoxide
toxicity.

305

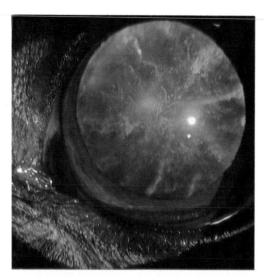

305 Secondary cataract to retinal disease—generalised progressive retinal atrophy (Miniature Poodle, 7 years old) The typical appearance of anterior and posterior cortical cataract.

306

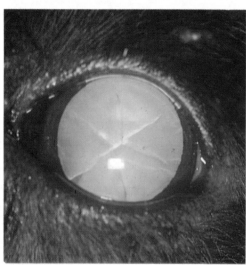

306 Secondary cataract to retinal disease—generalised progressive retinal atrophy (Miniature Poodle, 5 years old) Note the tapetal glow visible through the total cataract.

307

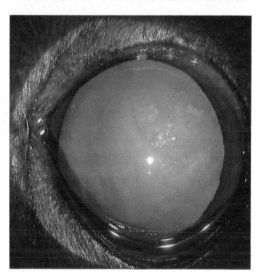

307 Secondary cataract to retinal disease—generalised progressive retinal atrophy (Miniature Poodle, 5 years old) Total dense and mature cataract.

308 Secondary cataract to central progressive retinal atrophy (Labrador, 10 years old)

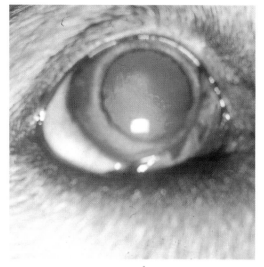

309 Secondary cataract to retinal dysplasia (English Springer Spaniel, 8 months old)

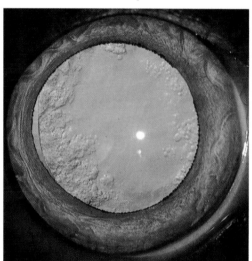

310 Cataract secondary to glaucoma (Border Collie, 5 years old) Note the congested blood vessels and dilated pupil.

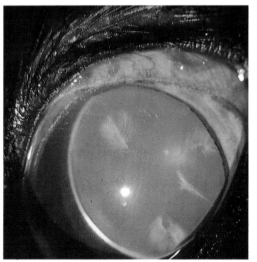

311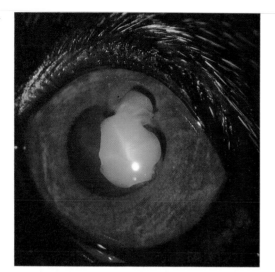

311 Traumatic cataract (Jack Russell Terrier, 2 years old) Note also uveitis and irregular pupil.

312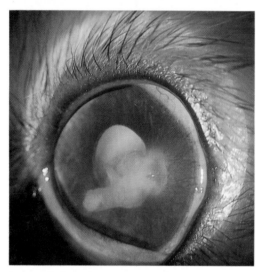

312 Traumatic cataract (Jack Russell Terrier, 4 months old) Note corneal puncture wound with blood vessels and lens material in the anterior chamber.

313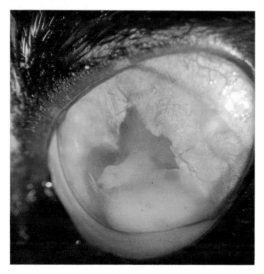

313 Traumatic cataract (DSH cat, 9 years old) A corneal wound, with uveitis and lens material in the anterior chamber.

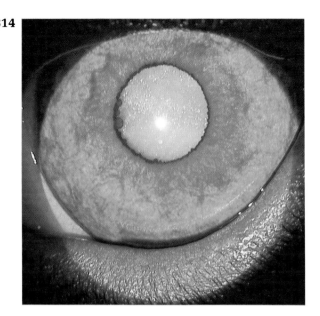

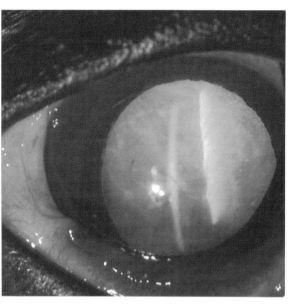

314 Resorbing cataract (English Springer Spaniel, 18 months old) Note the metallic appearance of the lens and pupillary cysts.

315 Resorbing cataract (American Cocker Spaniel, 18 months old) Note the slit-beam on the anterior lens capsule showing it to be flat and uneven.

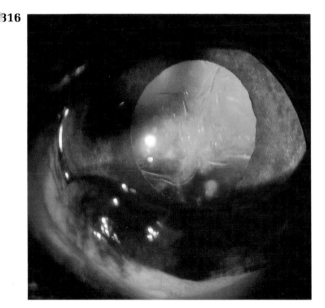

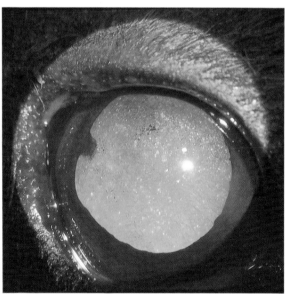

316 Resorbing cataract (Great Dane, 4 years old) Note the wrinkled anterior capsule.

317 Resorbing cataract (Lakeland Terrier) Green tapetal reflex and posterior synechiae (post-uveitis) at 9 o'clock.

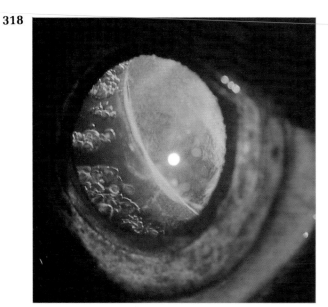

318 Cataract and posterior lenticonus (Labrador, 18 months old) Unilateral in this case.

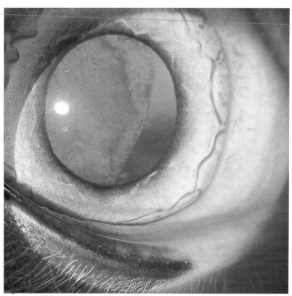

319 Cataract and coloboma (Old English Sheepdog, 3 months old) This case had multiple congenital ocular anomalies.

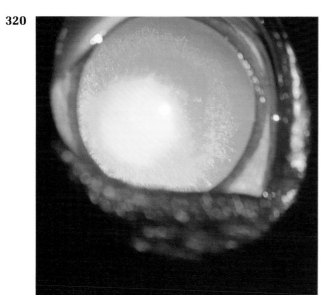

320 Cataract and hyaloid artery (Border Collie, young adult) *See also* **352** and **353**.

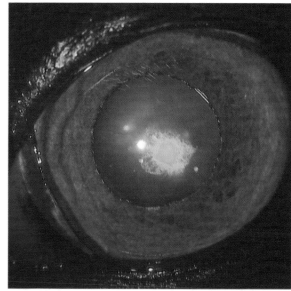

321 Anterior polar cataract (Lurcher, 6 years old) Bilateral in this case.

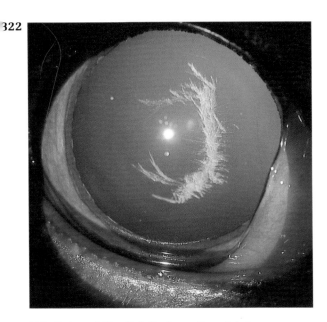

322 Cataract (English Springer Spaniel, 6 years old) Feather-like opacity around part of the edge of the nucleus (lamellar-type).

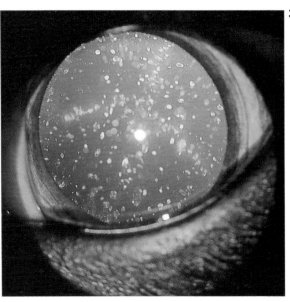

323 Cataract (Border Collie, 18 months old) Multiple, subcapsular focal dots particularly involving suture lines and bilateral.

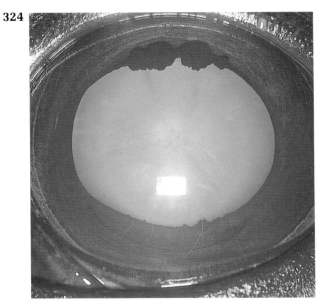

324 Total cataract (Thoroughbred, 5 years old) Mature cataract of unknown aetiology.

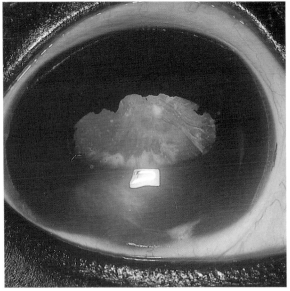

325 Partial cataract (Hunter, 7 years old) Traumatic cataract—note the corneal scar at 5 o'clock.

False Cataracts

326

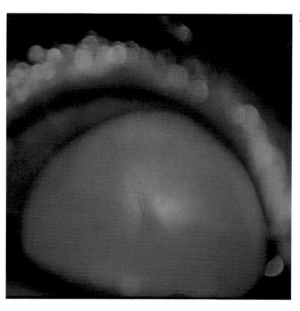

327

326 Temporary opacity (Miniature long-haired Dachshund, 13 weeks old) Opacities at ends of anterior suture line.

327 Temporary opacity (Shetland Sheepdog, 16 weeks old) Note appearance of lens fibres.

328

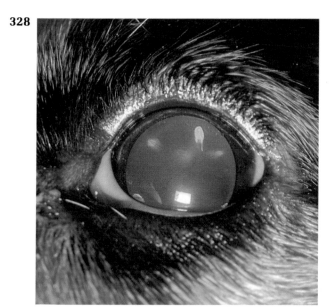

329

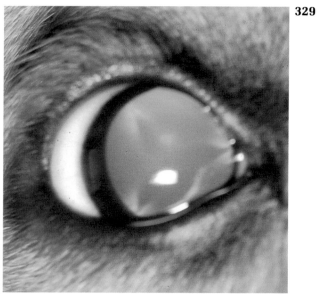

328 Temporary opacity (Beagle, 6 months old) Present on both anterior and posterior suture lines.

329 Temporary opacity (Cardigan Corgi puppy) A similar type but taking a different form.

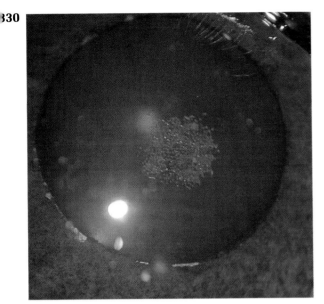

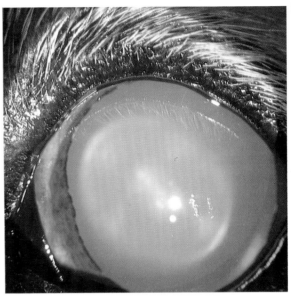

330 Pigment on anterior lens capsule (Cocker Spaniel, gold, 5 years old) Particularly common in this breed. It appears as a lens opacity by distant direct ophthalmoscopy.

331 Senile nuclear sclerosis (Labrador, 13 years old) The lens appears opalescent in direct light—a normal age change.

Lens Luxation

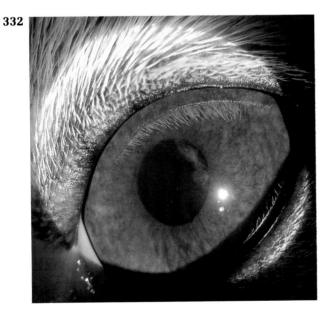

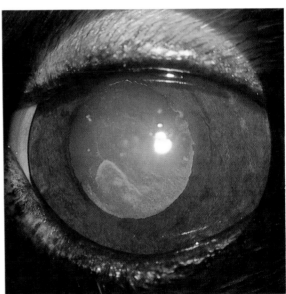

332 Vitreous in the pupil (Jack Russell Terrier, 4 years old) Note the appearance of vitreous on the right hand side of the pupil.

333 Vitreous in the pupil (Jack Russell Terrier, 5 years old) Note the swirling vitreous in front of the lens.

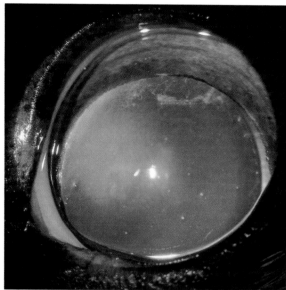

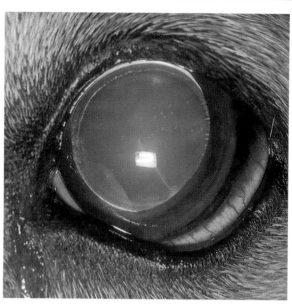

334 Anterior luxation (Border Collie) Lens dislocating through a dilated pupil—again note the vitreous.

335 Anterior luxation (Crossbred Terrier, 5 years old) Note the light on the superior edge of the lens as it passes through the pupil.

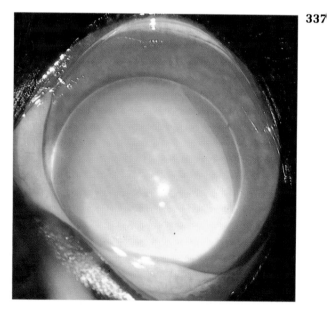

336 Anterior luxation (Sealyham, 4 years old) Lens completely through the pupil. Note the corneal opacity just below centre due to pressure of the lens on the corneal endothelium.

337 Anterior luxation (Wire-haired Fox Terrier, 4 years old) Note the distorted pupil due to the position of the lens, and the edge of the pupil visible through the lens.

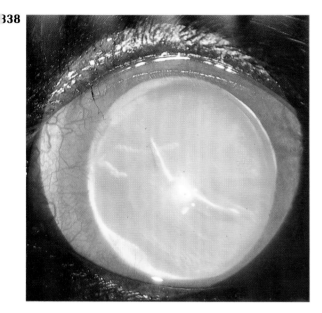

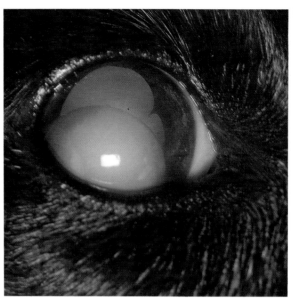

338 Anterior luxation (Jack Russell Terrier, 4 years old) Pupil block and secondary glaucoma.

339 Anterior luxation (Jack Russell Terrier, 4 years old) Anteriorly-dislocated lens becoming cataractous. Note the adhesion from pupil edge to lens capsule at 2 o'clock.

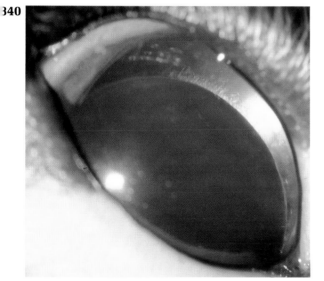

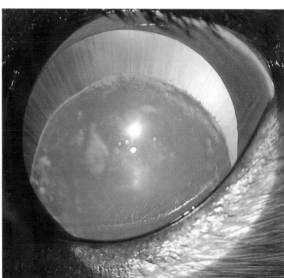

340 Aphakic crescent (Jack Russell Terrier, 5 years old) Note zonular fibres on the lens periphery.

341 Aphakic crescent (Shetland Sheepdog, 17 months old) Partial dislocation with stretching of the zonular fibres.

342

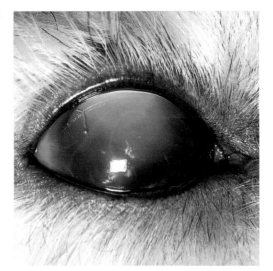

342 Posterior dislocation (Sealyham, 6 years old)
Aphakic, dilated pupil with the lens in the vitreous.

343

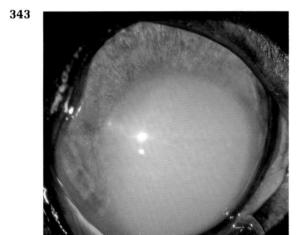

343 Posterior luxation (Jack Russell Terrier, 3 years old) Lens behind the iris but note the subcentral corneal oedema marking a previous anterior luxation.

344

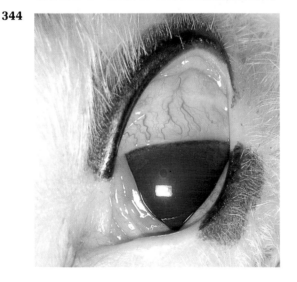

344 Secondary glaucoma (Sealyham Terrier, 5 years old) Note early conjunctival congestion.

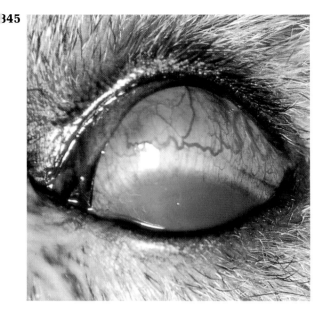

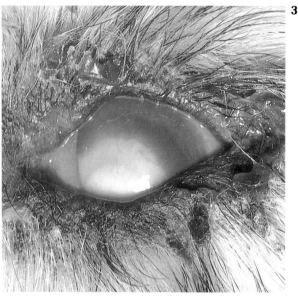

345 Secondary glaucoma (Welsh Terrier, 4 years old) Hydrophthalmos with scleral ectasia in the ciliary region.

346 Secondary glaucoma (Sealyham, 7 years old) Phthisis bulbi following hydrophthalmos.

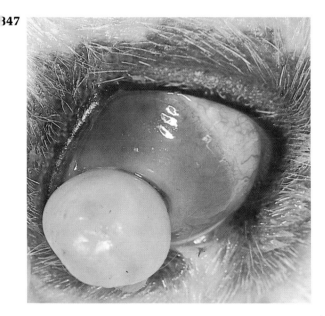

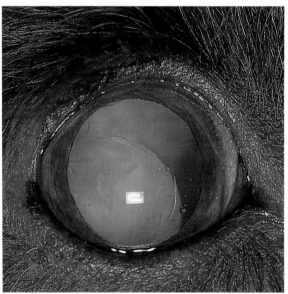

347 Extruded lens (Sealyham Terrier, 5 years old) Lens dislocated anteriorly and forced out through the cornea.

348 Dislocated cataract (Miniature Poodle, 8 years old) Posteriorly-dislocated cataractous lens. The primary condition was progressive retinal atrophy. Note the corneal clarity and the absence of clinical signs of glaucoma in this case of posterior luxation.

349

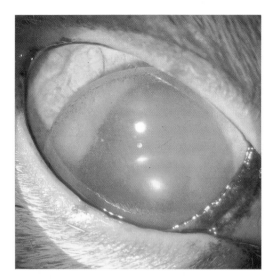

349 Anterior luxation (DSH cat, 10 years old) Lens luxation in this species is much less common than in the dog and usually occurs in aged animals.

350

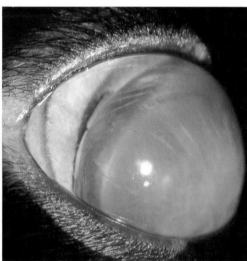

350 Anterior luxation (DSH cat, 10 years old)

351

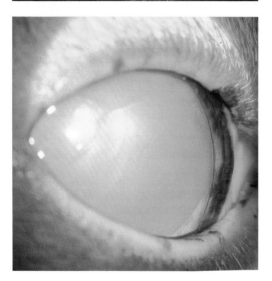

351 Dislocated cataract (DSH cat, 10 years old) Anteriorly-luxated cataract. Note the large size of the lens.

The Vitreous

Very little information is available at the moment on diseases affecting the vitreous body in the domestic animal. However, a number of conditions are illustrated and these include the congenital ones of persistent hyaloid remnant and artery, together with both hereditary and non-hereditary examples of persistent hyperplastic primary vitreous. In addition, the degenerative conditions with crystalline deposits (asteroid hyalosis and synchisis scintillans) and exogenous opacities (vitreal haemorrhage and cysts of two types) are shown.

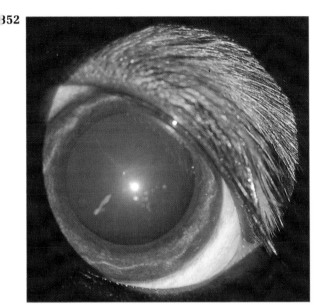

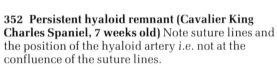

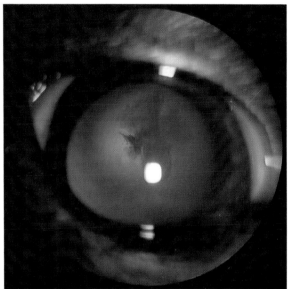

352 Persistent hyaloid remnant (Cavalier King Charles Spaniel, 7 weeks old) Note suture lines and the position of the hyaloid artery *i.e.* not at the confluence of the suture lines.

353 Persistent hyaloid artery (Shetland Sheepdog, 8 weeks old) Extensive hyaloid artery—this puppy also had optic disc colobomata (collie eye anomaly).

354 Synchisis scintillans (Golden Retriever, 11 years old) Associated extensive retinopathy is also present with liquefied vitreous.

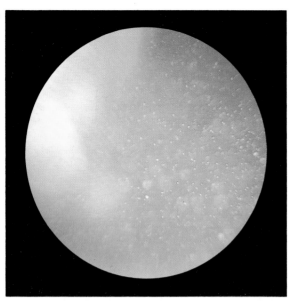

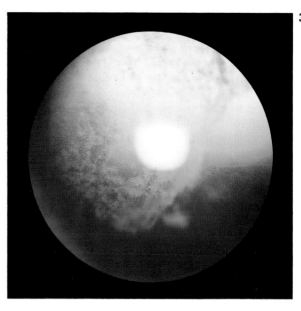

355 Asteroid hyalosis (Labrador cross, 6 years old) Particles in the vitreous do not move as in synchisis scintillans.

356 Hyalitis or syneresis (Labrador, 22 months old) Inflammation of the anterior vitreous of unknown aetiology.

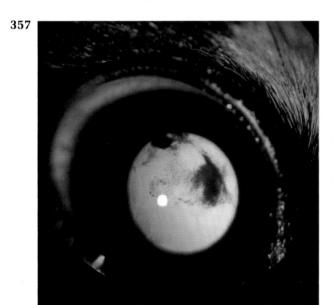

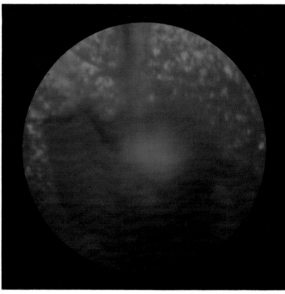

357 Vitreal haemorrhage (Chihuahua, 4 years old) Haemorrhage in the anterior vitreous. The cause is polycythaemia in this case.

358 Vitreal haemorrhage (English Springer Spaniel, 3 years old) Haemorrhage near the retina following shot in the eye.

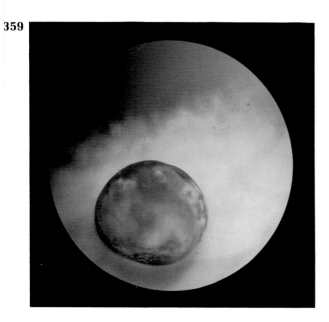

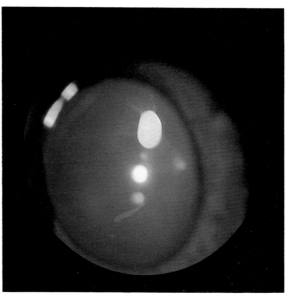

359 Cyst (Golden Retriever, 9 years old) Uveal cyst in front of the retina (*see also* **218**).

360 Cyst (Flat-coated Retriever, 2 years) Oval non-pigmented vitreal cyst.

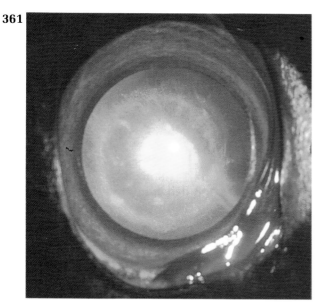

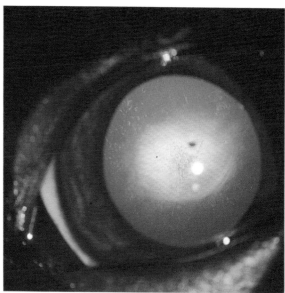

361 Persistent hyperplastic primary vitreous (Cocker Spaniel, 6 months old) Unilateral case showing large, persistent hyaloid artery, posterior plaque and vascular rete.

362 Persistent hyperplastic primary vitreous (Staffordshire Bull Terrier, 5 months old) Posterior plaque and persistent hyaloid artery. Bilateral and hereditary in this breed.

The Normal Canine Fundus

367

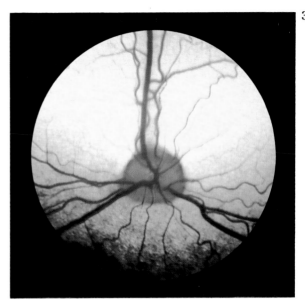

367 The fundus (Greyhound, young adult)
Posterior segment of the canine eye showing the
extent of the tapetal fundus (tapetum lucidum).

368

**368 The tapetum (Greyhound, young adult,
brindle)** Mainly yellow tapetal fundus with a green
and blue border.

369

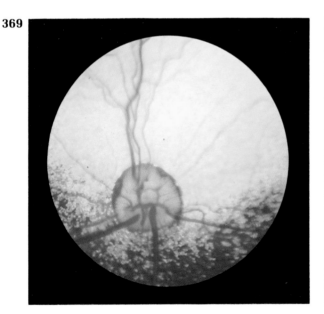

**369 The tapetum (Cocker Spaniel, 2 years old,
gold)** Yellow tapetal fundus.

370

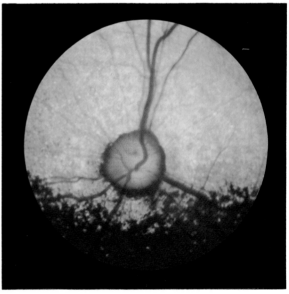

**370 The tapetum (Miniature Poodle, 1 year old,
black)** Green tapetal fundus.

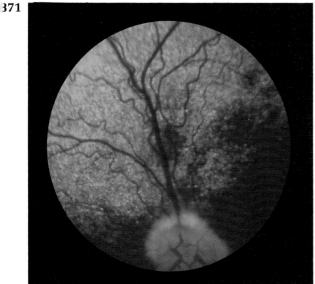

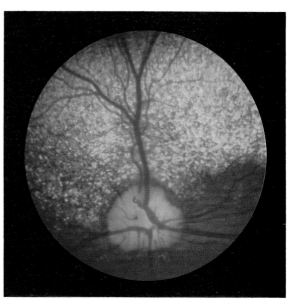

371 The tapetum (Boxer, 3 years old, red) Blue tapetal fundus.

372 The tapetum (Labrador, 1 year old, yellow) Sparsely scattered colours over a pale fawn background.

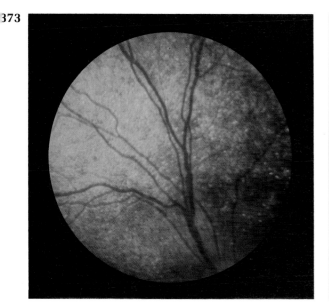

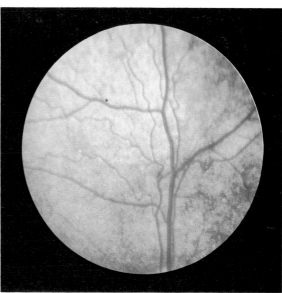

373 The tapetum (Shetland Sheepdog, 1 year old, merle) Sparsely scattered tapetal colours. *See also* **374** and **375, 386-391**.

374 The tapetum (Shetland Sheepdog, 5 years old, merle) Pale fawn fundus with a brown iris.

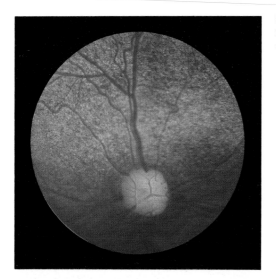

375 The tapetum (Shetland Sheepdog, 2 years old, merle) Similar to the previous figure with a poorly developed tapetum.

375

376

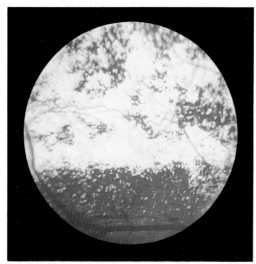

376 The tapetum (Border Collie, 1 year, tricolour) Breakup of the tapetal fundus by patches of tapetum nigrum.

377

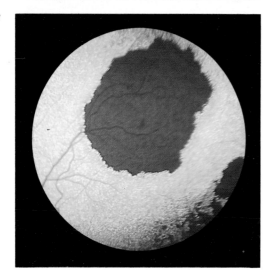

377 The tapetum (Golden Retriever, 6 years old) Demarcated island of tapetum nigrum within the tapetum lucidum area. Note the normal course of the retinal blood vessel.

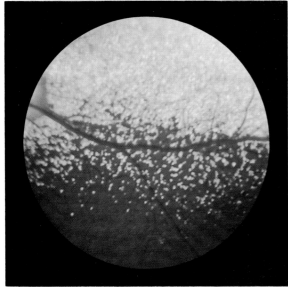

378 The tapetal junction (Golden Retriever, 4 years old) Gradual merging of tapetal into non-tapetal fundus.

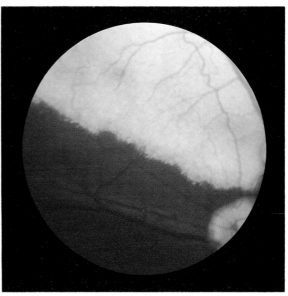

379 The tapetal junction (Pembroke Corgi, 10 months old, red) Sudden demarcation between the two areas. This situation is usually seen in short-coated dogs, whereas the previous figure illustrates the long-coated varieties.

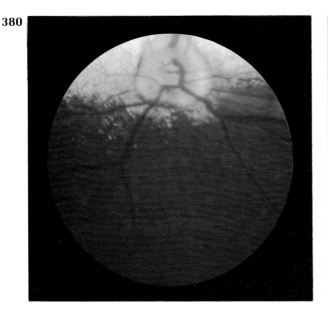

380 The tapetum nigrum (Greyhound, 4 years old, fawn) The usual appearance is of a dark grey-brown homogeneous region.

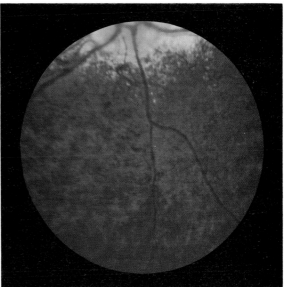

381 The tapetum nigrum (Labrador, 4 years old, yellow) The upper non-tapetal fundus may be more brown and paler than below.

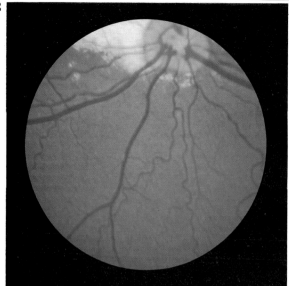

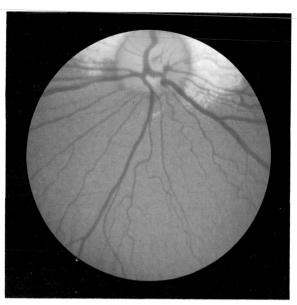

382 The tapetum nigrum (Labrador, 1 year old, chocolate) The non-tapetal fundus in dogs of this, or similar, coat colour (brown, chocolate, liver) is less heavily pigmented and appears paler, or as in the following figure.

383 The tapetum nigrum (Pointer, 3 years old, liver) Choroidal vascular pattern producing tigroid non-tapetal fundus.

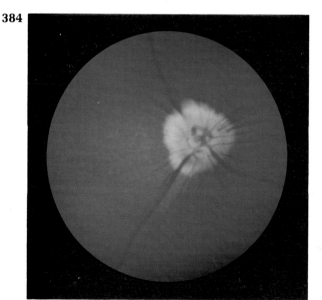

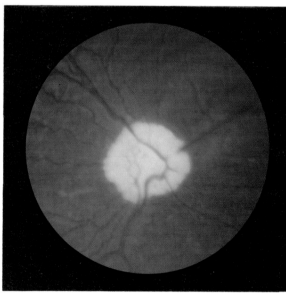

384 Red fundus (Beagle, 9 months old, tricolour) Known as 'ruby eye'—the iris was pale lemon in colour.

385 Absence of tapetum (Boston Terrier, 8 years old, brindle) Absence of any tapetal development.

386 Subalbinotic fundus (Shetland Sheepdog, 3 years old, merle, pale blue iris) Absence of a tapetum and appearance of choroidal vessels superimposed on the scleral background throughout the fundus.

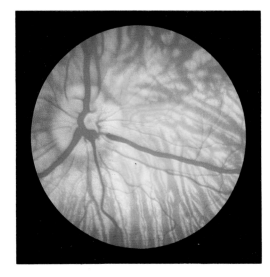

387 Subalbinotic fundus (Shetland Sheepdog, 2 years old, merle) Similar to the previous figure.

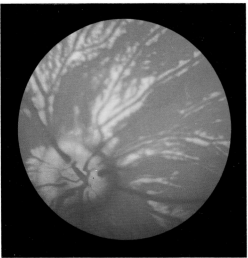

388 Subalbinotic fundus (Shetland Sheepdog, 1 year old, merle) Note the absence of a tapetum and a segment of subalbinism at 2 o'clock.

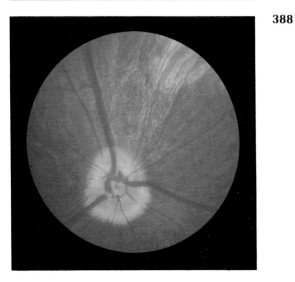

389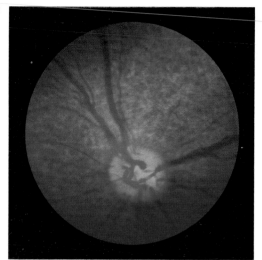

389 Subalbinotic fundus (Shetland Sheepdog, 5 months old, merle) Subalbinism, peripapillary and above the disc.

390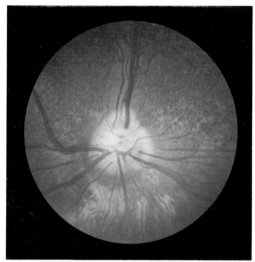

390 Subalbinotic fundus (Rough Collie, 1 year old, merle) Subalbinism below the disc.

391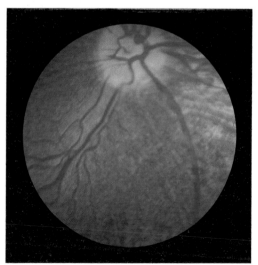

391 Subalbinotic fundus (Shetland Sheepdog, 10 months old, merle) Similar to the previous figure. Note the haphazard distribution of areas of subalbinism in the normal fundus of **386-391** and compare with the pathological chorioretinal dysplasia in collie eye anomaly (**498-506**).

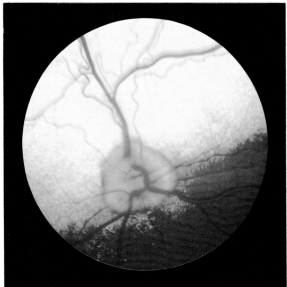

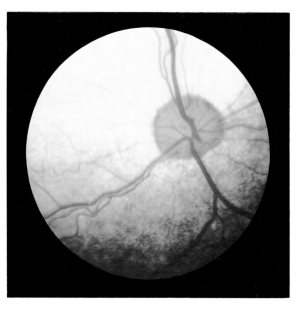

392 The optic disc (Greyhound, young adult, fawn)
The common position of the disc is just inside the
tapetum lucidum.

393 The optic disc (Labrador, 7 months old, yellow)
Occasionally it may appear completely inside the
tapetal fundus.

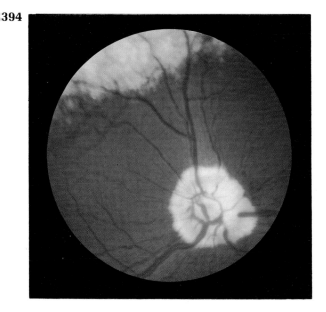

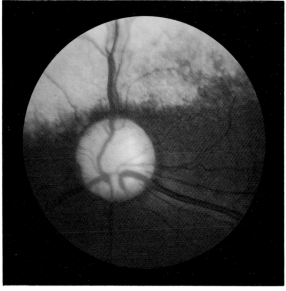

**394 The optic disc (Crossbred, 6 years old, black
and tan)** Occasionally it may appear inside the
non-tapetal fundus—these positions simply reflect
the extent of the tapetal fundus.

**395 The optic disc (Miniature Long-haired
Dachshund, 10 months old, black and tan)** There is
considerable variation in size from large to small
(see next figure).

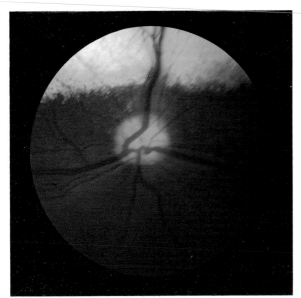

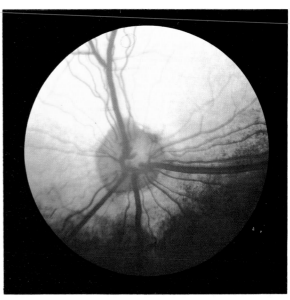

396 The optic disc (Beagle, 10 months old, tricolour) Micropapilla—normal variant. Compare with pathological optic nerve hypoplasia (**618** and **619**).

397 The optic disc (German Shepherd Dog, 1 year old) Variations in colour range from deep pink to white (as shown in the next figure).

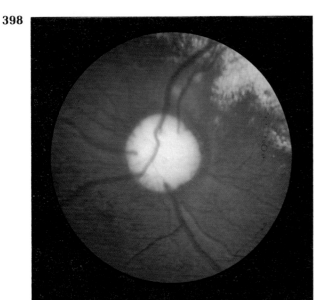

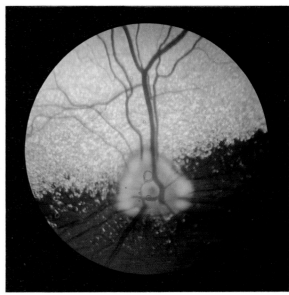

398 The optic disc (Chihuahua, 4 years old, black and tan) Pale disc but note normal retinal blood vessels. Compare with optic atrophy (**613** and **614**).

399 The optic disc (Briard, 5 years old, black) Physiological pit—small grey spot in centre of disc.

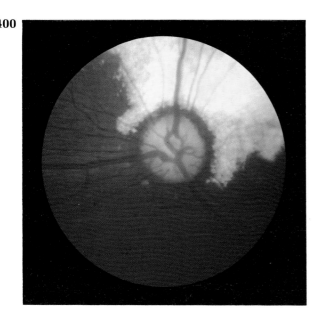

400 The optic disc (Yorkshire Terrier, 1 year old, black and tan) Partial pigmented ring to the disc.

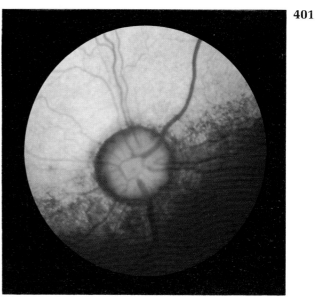

401 The optic disc (Beagle, 6 months old, tricolour) Complete pigmented ring to disc.

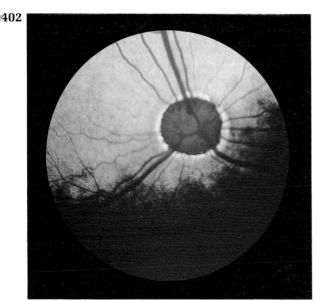

402 The optic disc (Labrador, 1 year old, black) Reflective ring to disc, or conus.

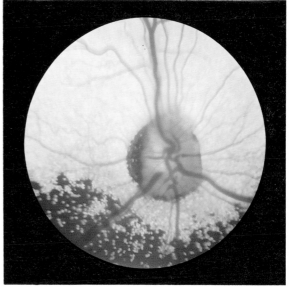

403 The optic disc (Golden Retriever, 2 years old) The shape of the disc varies very much in the dog. In this figure the disc is oval with a pigmented area on one side.

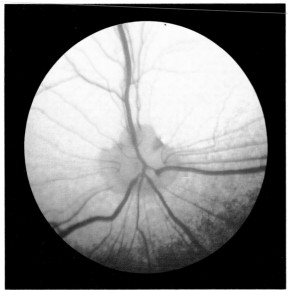

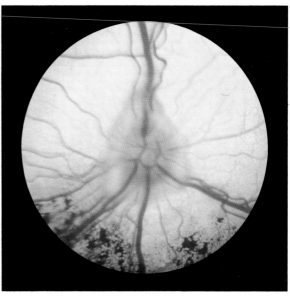

404 The optic disc (German Shepherd Dog, 2 years old, black and tan) Shamrock shape.

405 The optic disc (German Shepherd Dog, 10 months old) Large disc due to medullated fibres—pseudopapilloedema.

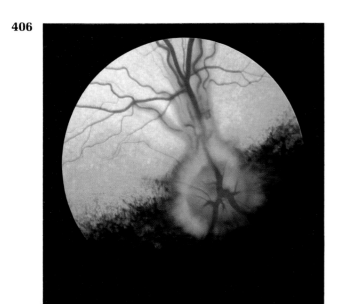

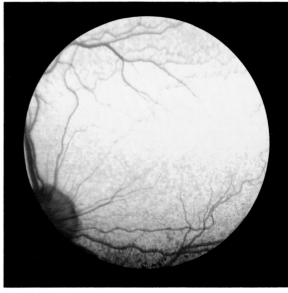

406 The optic disc (German Shepherd Dog, 1 year old) Medullated fibres extending away from the disc.

407 Retinal blood vessels (English Springer Spaniel, 2 years old) Well-developed vascular pattern above and below the area centralis.

408 Retinal blood vessels (Border Collie, 1 year old, black and white) Four primary veins.

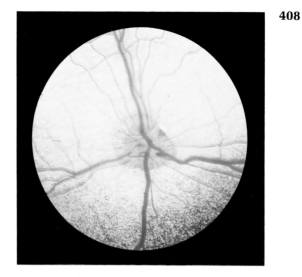

409 Retinal blood vessels (Rough Collie, 1 year old, tricolour) Note the tortuosity of the retinal arterioles (normal, not excessive).

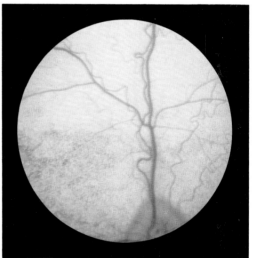

410 Retinal blood vessels (English Springer Spaniel, 2 years old, liver and white) Unusual vascular pattern.

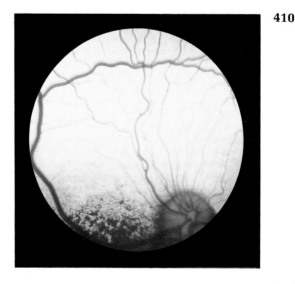

Development of the Canine Fundus

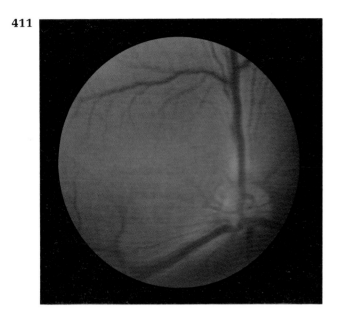

411 Very early appearance with no differentiation into tapetal and non-tapetal fundus

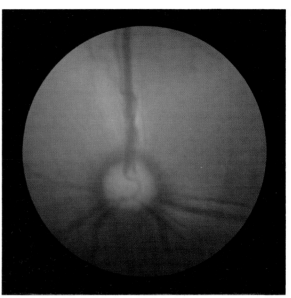

412 Greyhound puppy, 23 days old

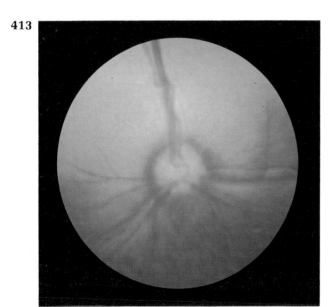

413 Greyhound puppy, 27 days old

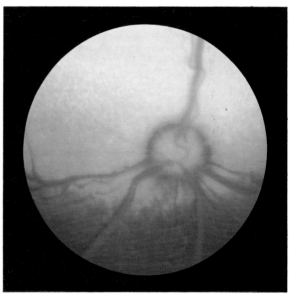

414 Greyhound puppy, 51 days old

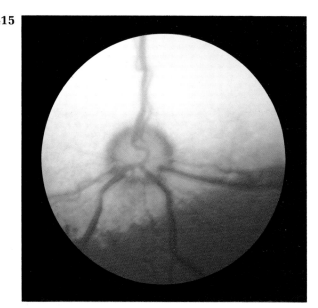

415 Greyhound puppy, 58 days old

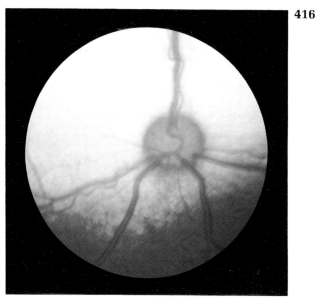

416 Greyhound puppy, 65 days old

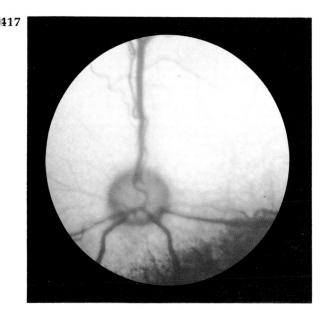

417 Greyhound puppy, 3 months old

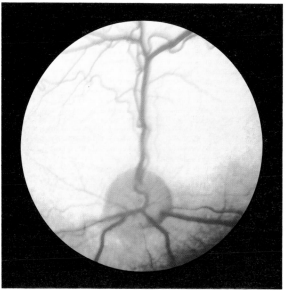

418 Greyhound puppy, 6 months old Normal adult
appearance.

The Normal Feline Fundus

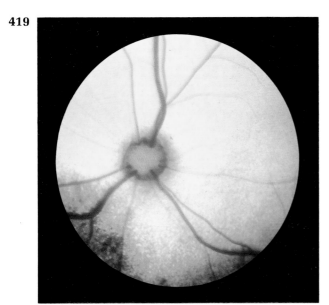

419 Yellow tapetum (DSH cat)

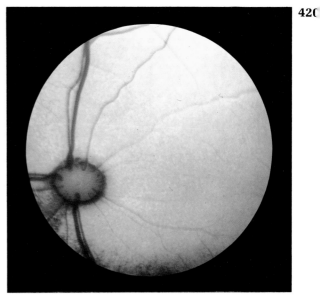

420 Yellow green tapetum (DSH cat)

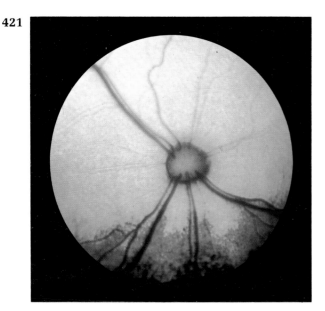

421 Yellow green tapetum (DSH cat)

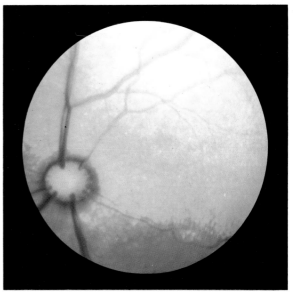

422 Blue green tapetum (DSH cat)

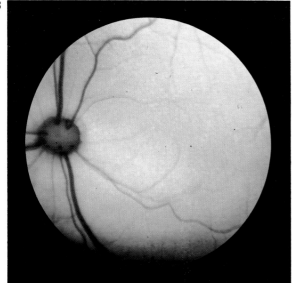

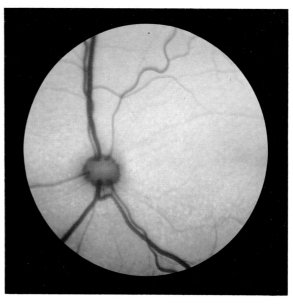

423 Vascular pattern (DSH cat) Note the blood vessels surrounding the area centralis.

424 Area centralis (DSH cat) Note the region lateral and immediately opposite the optic disc.

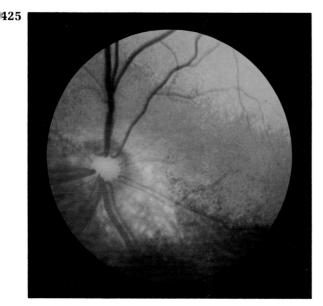

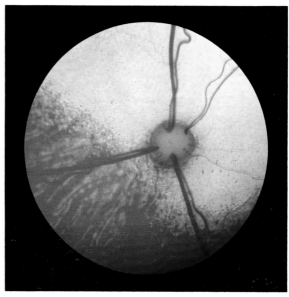

425 Subalbinism (DSH cat)

426 Tigroid tapetum nigrum (Siamese cat, 2 years old, seal-point) Tigroid non-tapetal fundus.

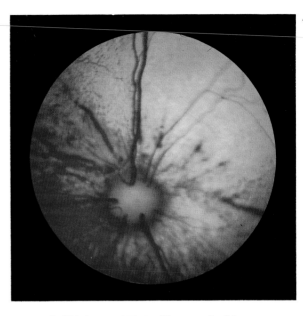

42

427 Subalbinism (DSH cat, blue-eyed white, young adult) Note appearance and colours of tapetal and non-tapetal fundus.

428 Subalbinism (DSH cat, blue-eyed white, young adult) Note appearance and colours of tapetal and non-tapetal fundus.

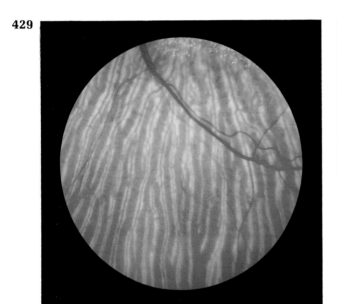

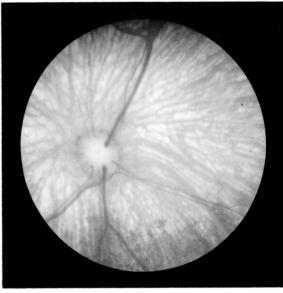

43

429 Subalbinism (DSH cat, blue-eyed white, young adult) Choroidal vessels in non-tapetal fundus region.

430 Subalbinism of the whole fundus (DSH cat, blue-eyed white, young adult)

The Normal Equine Fundus

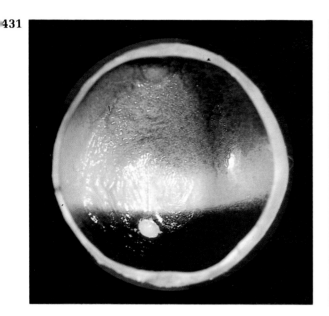

431 The ocular fundus (Thoroughbred adult)
Posterior segment of the equine eye showing the
extent of the tapetal fundus. Compare with **367**.

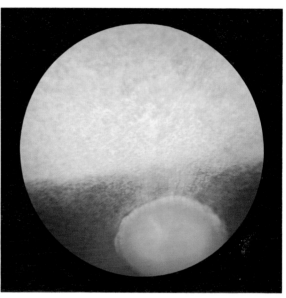

432 The tapetum (Hunter-type, 6 years old, black)
Yellow green tapetal fundus.

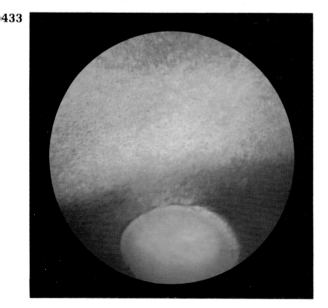

433 The tapetum (Hunter-type, 6 years old, grey)

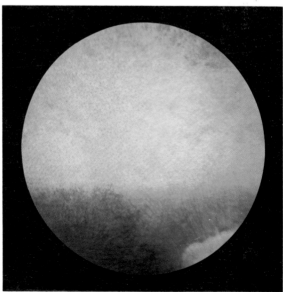

**434 The tapetum (Welsh pony, 7 years old, blue
roan)** Two-coloured, due to the thickness of the
tapetum.

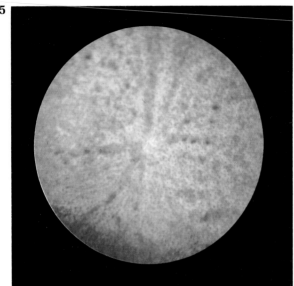

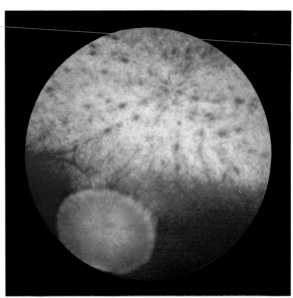

435 The tapetum (Thoroughbred, 4 years old, chestnut) Pattern due to underlying choroidal vessels.

436 The tapetum (Welsh pony, 1 year old, skewbald) Similar pattern to the previous figure, with heterochromic iris.

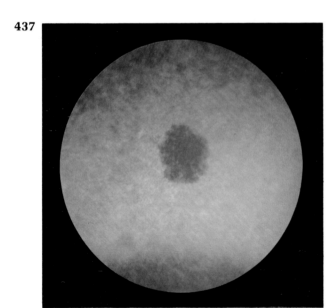

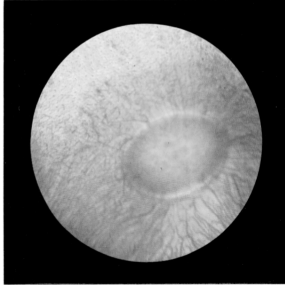

437 The tapetum (Hunter-type, 6 years old, grey) Non-tapetal island within the tapetal fundus.

438 Subalbinism (Palomino x albino pony, 8 months, white) Note the poorly-developed tapetum and visible choroidal vessels in the non-tapetal fundus.

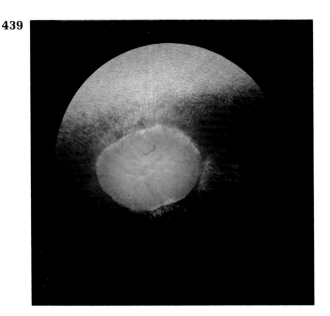

439 Tapetum nigrum (Arab, 8 years old, grey) Note the lack of pigment immediately superior to the disc.

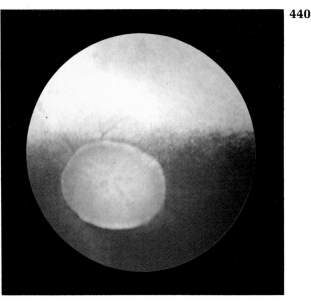

440 The optic disc (Thoroughbred, 9 years old, bay) Large pale disc adjacent to the tapetal fundus.

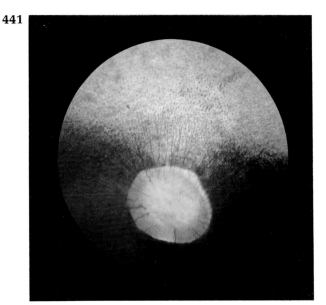

441 The optic disc (Shetland pony, 4 years old, brown) Small irregular shaped disc.

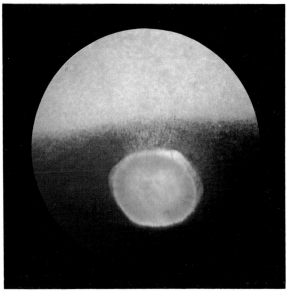

442 The optic disc (Thoroughbred, 1 year old, chestnut) Disc inside the non-tapetal fundus and with a double edge in places.

443

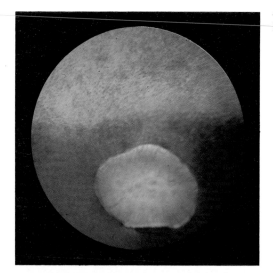

443 The optic disc (pony, 15 years old, skewbald)
Dark red disc with heavy pigment along the base.

444

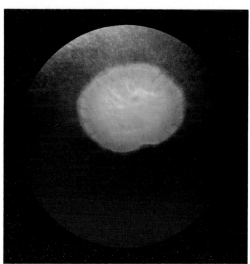

444 The optic disc (Thoroughbred, 3 years old, chestnut) Indentation along lower border of disc.

445

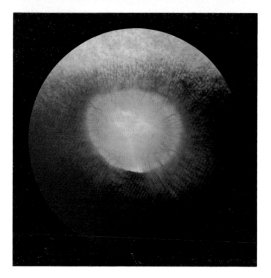

445 The optic disc (Thoroughbred, 1 year old, bay)
Medullated nerve fibres around the disc giving a halo effect.

446 The optic disc (Welsh pony, 8 years old, roan)
Medullated nerve fibres, particularly at the inferior lateral angle.

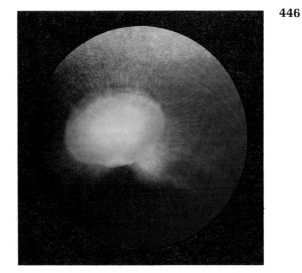

446

447 The fundus (Thoroughbred foal, 1 day old)
Note the similarity to the adult fundus in this species. Compare with **411-418** in the dog.

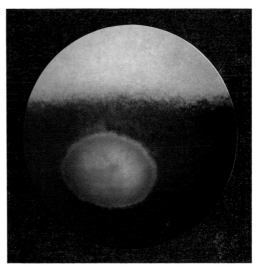

447

448 The fundus (donkey, young adult)

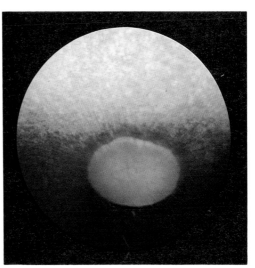

448

The Normal Bovine and Ovine Fundus

449

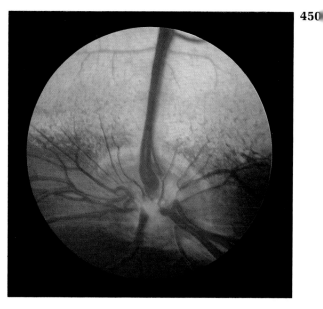

449 The fundus (Shorthorn calf) Note the obvious difference between artery and vein.

450

450 The fundus (Shorthorn calf) Note the conus vestigialis in the centre of the disc.

451

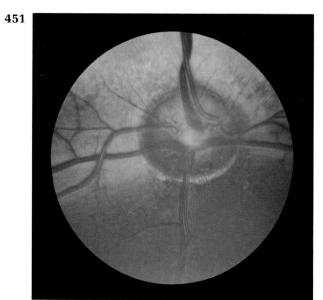

451 The fundus (Jersey cow) Note the dark colour of the disc.

452

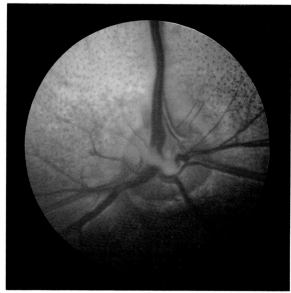

452 The fundus (Charolais calf)

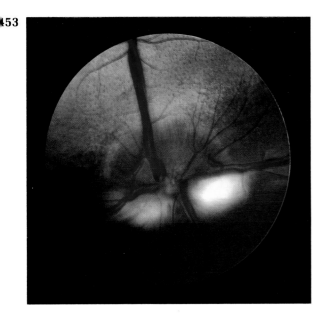

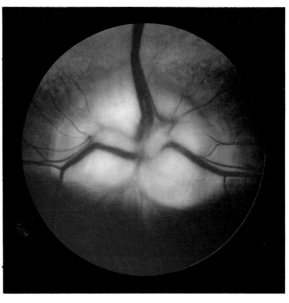

453 Optic disc (Friesian cow) Medullated fibres of the optic disc at the base.

454 Optic disc (Friesian cow) Medullated fibres of optic disc.

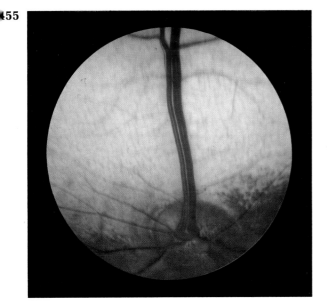

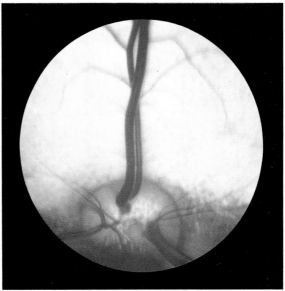

455 Sheep fundus (adult ewe)

456 Sheep fundus (adult ewe)

457

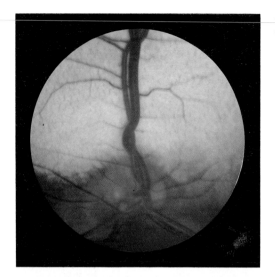

457 Sheep fundus (Crossbred Hill sheep, adult ewe)

458

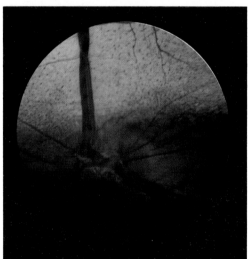

458 Sheep fundus (Clun cross, adult ewe)
Non-medullated optic disc fibres.

459

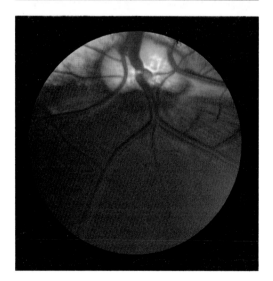

459 Sheep fundus (adult ewe) Note the medullated fibres from the disc and the appearance of the non-tapetal fundus.

Other Animals

460 Human (young adult female) Note macula.

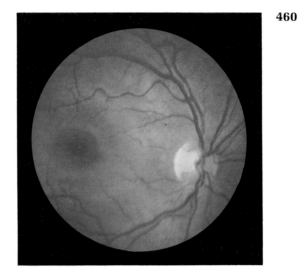

461 Monkey (young adult baboon) Note macula.

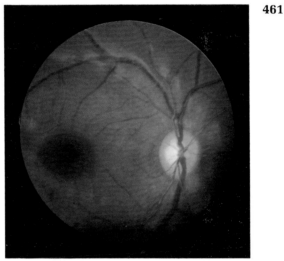

462 Rabbit (Albino, young adult)

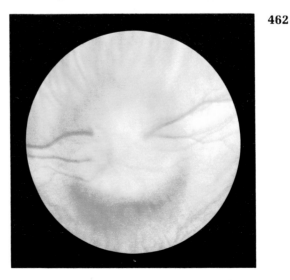

463

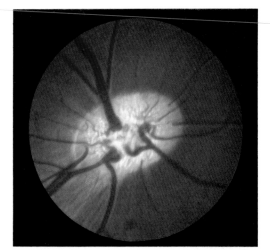

463 Pig (young adult) Note the absence of a tapetum.

464

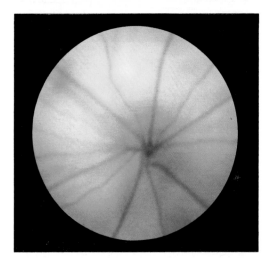

464 Rat (young adult)

465

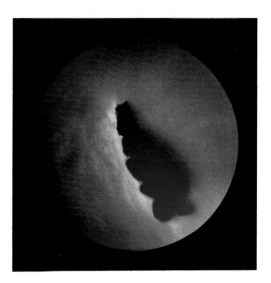

465 Bird (Tawny Owl) Note pecten.

Generalised Progressive Retinal Atrophy

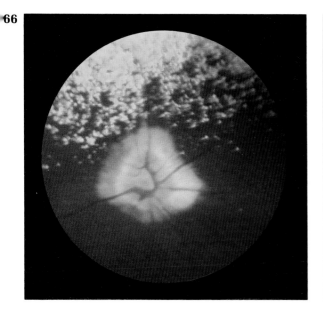
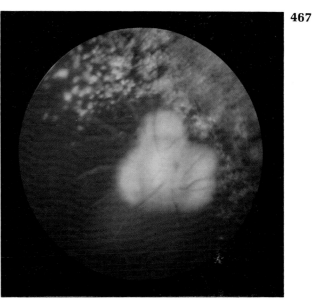

466 Rod-cone degeneration (Miniature Poodle, 5 years old, black) Note the narrowed retinal blood vessels.

467 Rod-cone degeneration (Miniature Poodle, 8 years old, black) Advanced degeneration with pale disc and visible choroidal vessels.

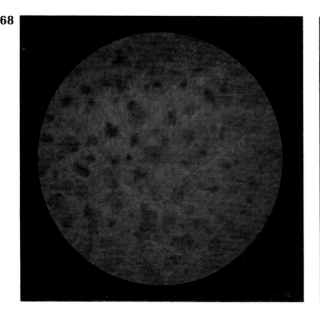
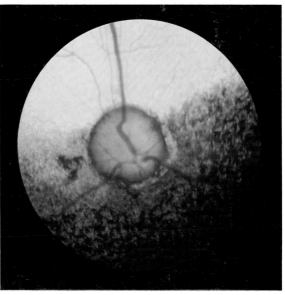

468 Rod-cone degeneration (Miniature Poodle, 5 years old, black) Typical appearance of the non-tapetal fundus.

469 Rod-cone degeneration (Cocker Spaniel, 2 years old, tricolour) Early ophthalmoscopic changes.

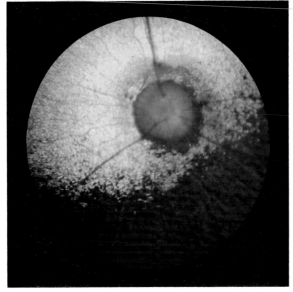

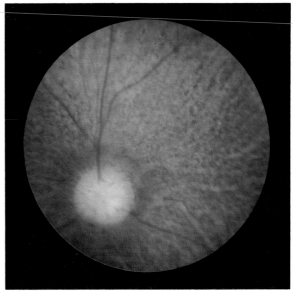

470 Rod-cone degeneration (Cocker Spaniel, 4 years old, blue roan) Right eye showing obvious ophthalmoscopic signs of narrowed blood vessels and increased tapetal reflectivity.

471 Rod-cone degeneration (Cocker Spaniel, 4 years old, blue roan) Left eye of the same dog as shown in the previous figure showing less obvious ophthalmoscopic signs due to subalbinism and the absence of the tapetum.

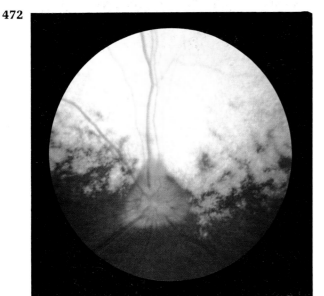

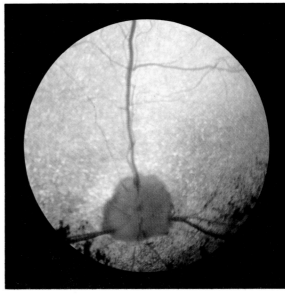

472 Rod dysplasia cone degeneration (Elkhound, 20 months old)

473 Progressive retinal atrophy (Tibetan Terrier, 18 months old)

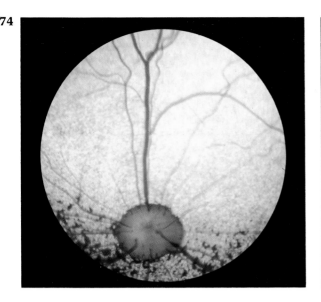

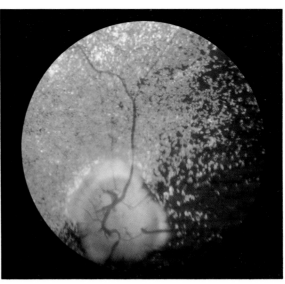

474 Progressive retinal atrophy (Tibetan Terrier, 15 months old) Early ophthalmoscopic signs.

475 Progressive retinal atrophy (Tibetan Spaniel, 4 years old)

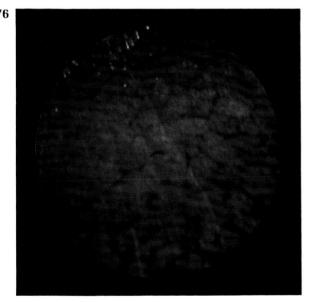

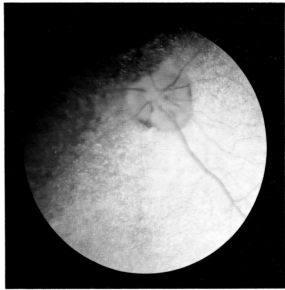

476 Progressive retinal atrophy (Tibetan Spaniel, 4 years old) Changes in non-tapetal fundus.

477 Progressive retinal atrophy (English Springer Spaniel, 21 months old, liver and white) Note the typical increased tapetal reflectivity.

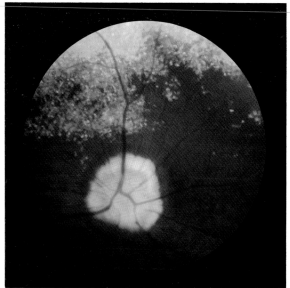

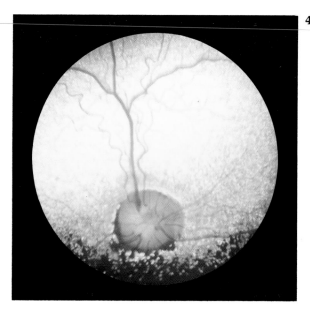

47

478 Progressive retinal atrophy (Miniature Schnauzer, 4 years old)

479 Rod-cone dysplasia (Irish Setter, 3 months old)

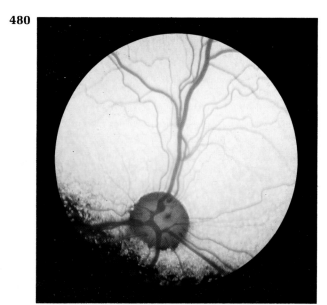

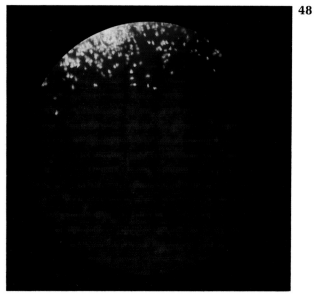

48

480 Normal fundus (Irish Setter, 3 months old)
Litter-mate to the animal seen in the previous figure, showing an obvious difference on comparison.

481 Rod-cone dysplasia (Irish Setter, 3 months old)
Changes in non-tapetal fundus.

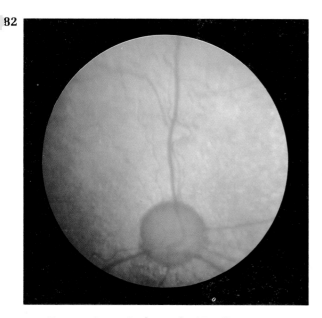

482 Progressive retinal atrophy (Cardigan Corgi, 3 months old)

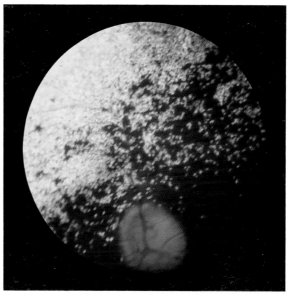

483 Progressive retinal atrophy (Miniature Long-haired Dachshund, 17 months old) An advanced case.

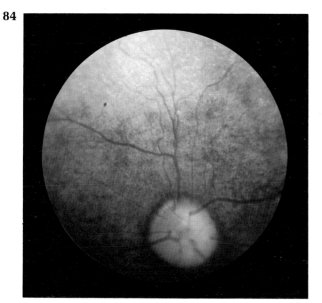

484 Progressive retinal atrophy (Miniature Long-haired Dachshund, 12 months old) Poor differentiation of the tapetum but obvious blood vessel attenuation.

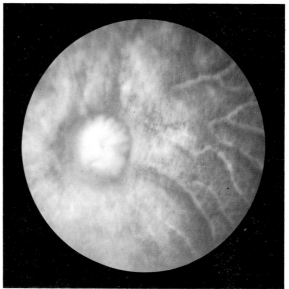

485 Progressive retinal atrophy (Miniature Long-haired Dachshund, 3 years old) Very advanced case.

Central Progressive Retinal Atrophy (Pigment Epithelial Dystrophy)

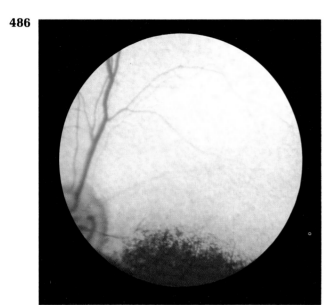

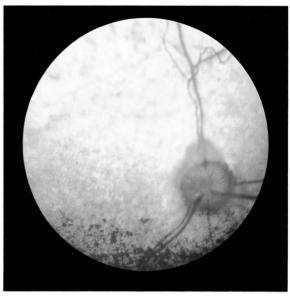

486 Labrador Retriever, 2 years old Note the early change in the area centralis.

487 Labrador Retriever, 4 years old Note the pigmentary change in the tapetal fundus.

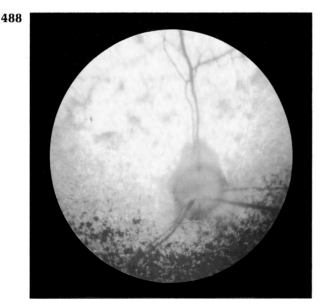

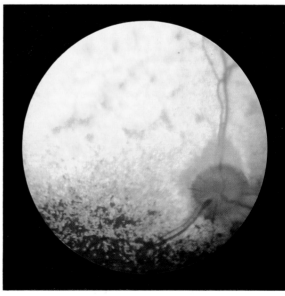

488 Labrador Retriever, 5 years old Same dog as in previous figure but one year later.

489 Labrador Retriever, 6 years old Same dog as in the previous two figures demonstrating the progressive nature of this retinopathy.

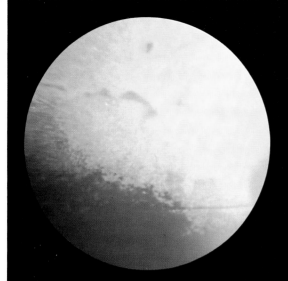

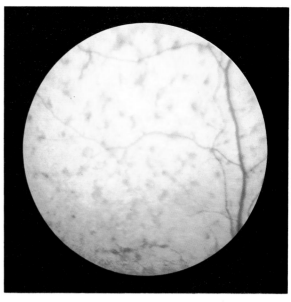

490 Labrador Retriever, 10 years old Advanced stage with fewer and denser pigment spots.

491 Labrador Retriever, 5 years old Note the pigmentation along the course of the retinal blood vessels.

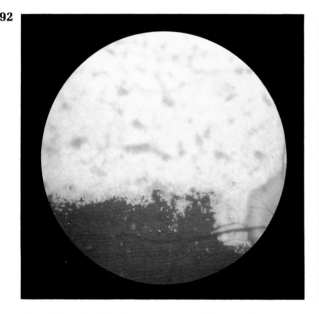

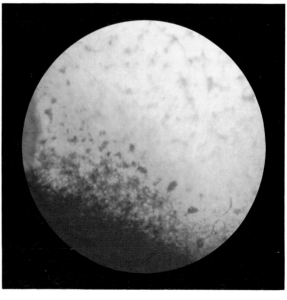

492 Labrador Retriever, 6 years old Note the increased tapetal reflectivity between the pigment spots.

493 Labrador Retriever, 4 years old Note the difference in the form of the pigment spots from the previous two figures.

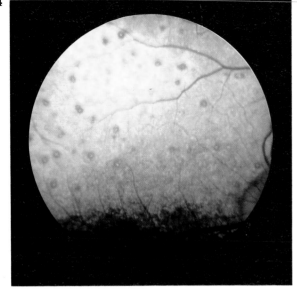

494 Labrador Retriever, 3 years old Note the cystic appearance of the pigment spots.

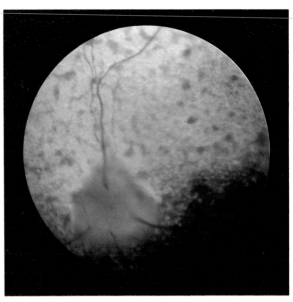

495 Border Collie, 6 years old

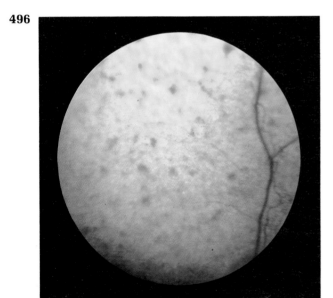

496 Rough Collie, 5 years old

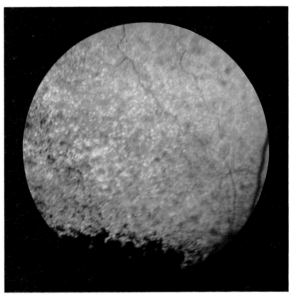

497 Briard, 8 years old

Collie Eye Anomaly

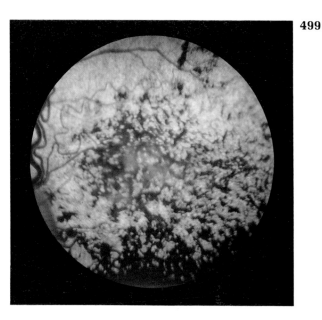

498 Chorioretinal dysplasia (Border Collie, 4 years old) Note the mild change in the area lateral to the optic disc.

499 Chorioretinal dysplasia (Border Collie, 4 years old) A more severe change in the eye of a litter-sister of the animal shown in **498**.

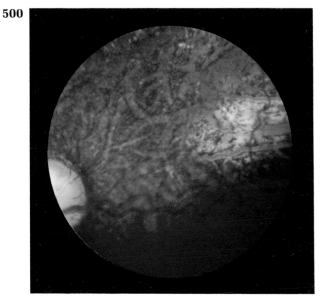

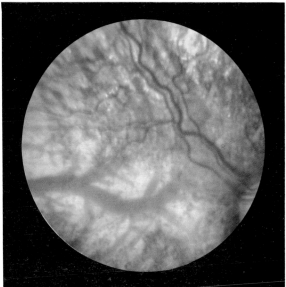

500 Chorioretinal dysplasia (Shetland Sheepdog, 7 months old) A more severe change than in the previous figure but in a similar position ie lateral to the optic disc.

501 Chorioretinal dysplasia (Rough Collie, 1 year old) A severe lesion adjacent to the disc.

502

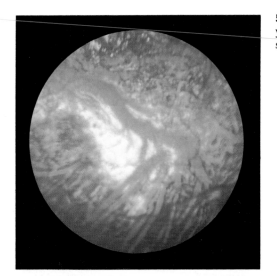

502 Chorioretinal dysplasia (Shetland Sheepdog, 2 years old) A severe lesion away from the disc but still in the typical position.

503

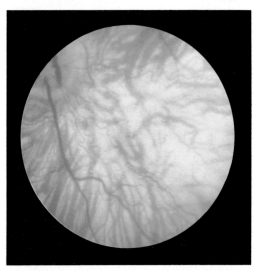

503 Chorioretinal dysplasia (Rough Collie, 2 years old, blue merle) The appearance of the lesion in a subalbinotic fundus.

504

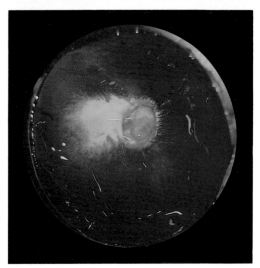

504 Chorioretinal dysplasia (Border Collie, 2 years old) Posterior segment of the eye showing a 'pale patch' (dysplastic area) opposite the optic disc. Note also the coloboma of the optic disc.

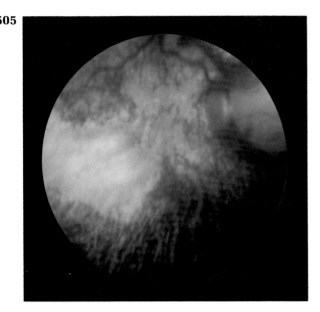

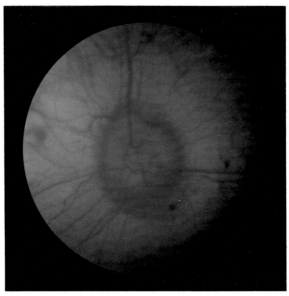

505 Chorioretinal dysplasia (Rough Collie, 8 weeks old) The appearance of the lesion in a young puppy.

506 Chorioretinal dysplasia (Shetland Sheepdog, 3 years old, blue merle) Extensive chorioretinal dysplasia in a subalbinotic fundus.

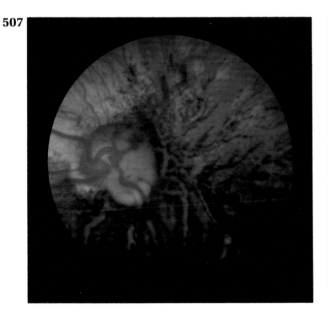

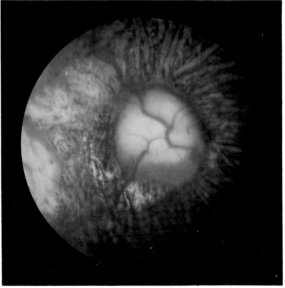

507 Coloboma (Rough Collie, 1 year old, blue merle) Small deep coloboma at 12 o'clock, together with chorioretinal dysplasia.

508 Coloboma (Shetland Sheepdog, 3 years old, sable) Shallow coloboma of the lower part of the optic disc, together with chorioretinal dysplasia.

509

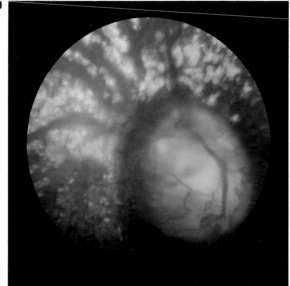

509 Coloboma (Border Collie, 3 years old, black and white) Medium-sized coloboma in the centre of the disc together with chorioretinal dysplasia.

510

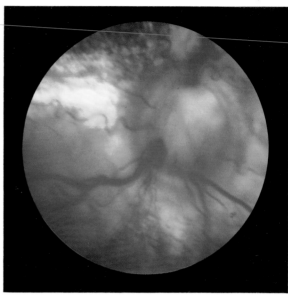

510 Coloboma (Rough Collie, 7 years old, blue merle) Large disc coloboma together with chorioretinal dysplasia and retinal detachment.

511

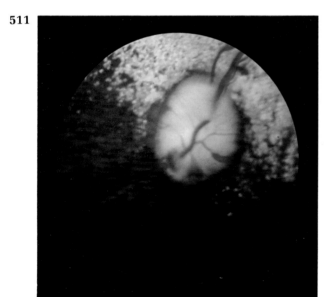

511 Coloboma (Shetland Sheepdog, 4 years old, sable) Two small colobomas at 6 o'clock together with mild chorioretinal dysplasia.

512

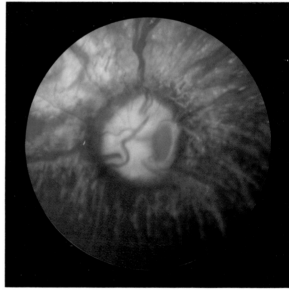

512 Coloboma (Shetland Sheepdog, 2 years old, sable) Coloboma in atypical position at 3 o'clock together with chorioretinal dysplasia.

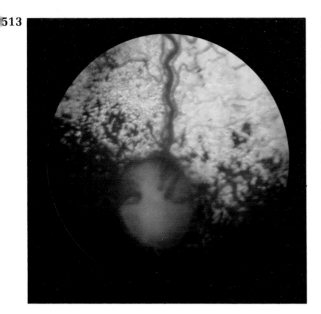

513 Coloboma (Rough Collie, 1 year old, tricolour)
Medium-sized coloboma of the ventral disc.

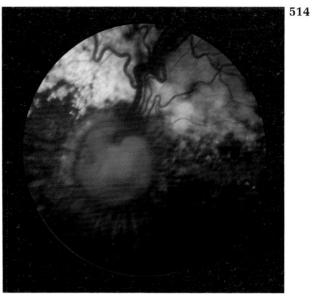

514 Coloboma (Shetland Sheepdog, 16 months old, sable) A whole disc coloboma together with chorioretinal dysplasia and retinal detachment in the upper right quadrant.

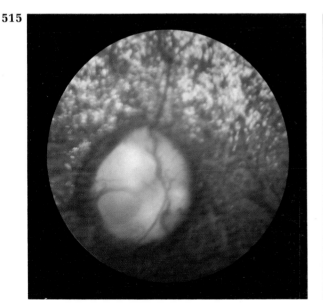

515 Coloboma (Shetland Sheepdog, 3 years old, tricolour) A shallow disc coloboma at 7 o'clock.

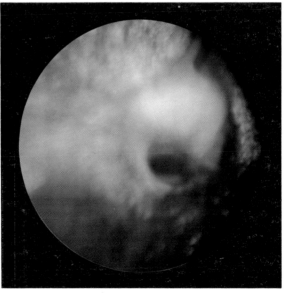

516 Coloboma (Shetland Sheepdog, 9 months old, sable) A deep disc coloboma at 7 o'clock.

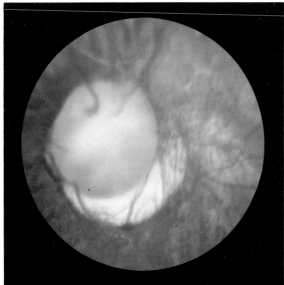

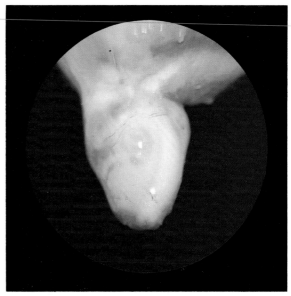

51

517 Coloboma (Shetland Sheepdog, 3 years old, tricolour) Large disc coloboma and adjacent peripapillary coloboma of the retina and choroid.

518 Coloboma (Rough Collie, 6 months old, sable) External appearance of optic disc coloboma—note cystic appearance and optic nerve reflected on right hand side.

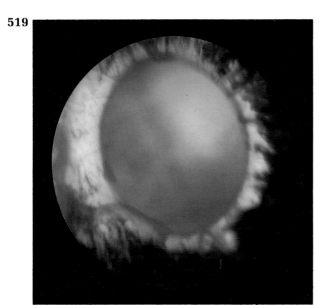

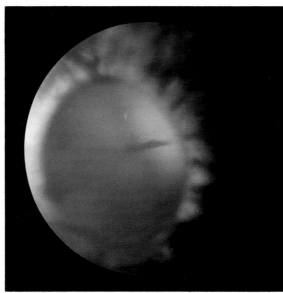

52

519 Coloboma (Shetland Sheepdog, 13 weeks old, tricolour) An extensive disc coloboma.

520 Coloboma (Shetland Sheepdog, 13 weeks old, tricolour) Same as the previous figure but focused to show the persistent hyaloid remnant; frequently found in conjunction with colobomata in all species (see also **635**).

521 Retinal detachment (Rough Collie, 1 year old, tricolour) Flat retinal detachment to the left of the optic disc.

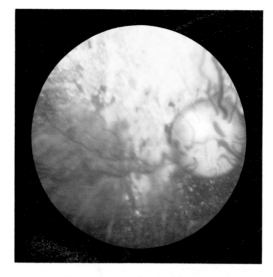

522 Retinal detachment (Shetland Sheepdog, 3 months old, sable) Extensive retinal detachment—note the tortuosity of the blood vessels.

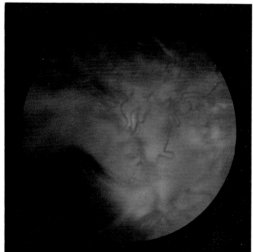

523 Retinal detachment (Shetland Sheepdog, 9 months old, blue merle) Extensive retinal detachment—note coloboma of the optic disc.

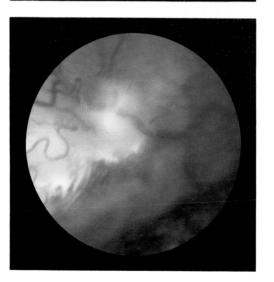

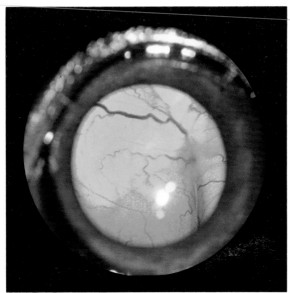

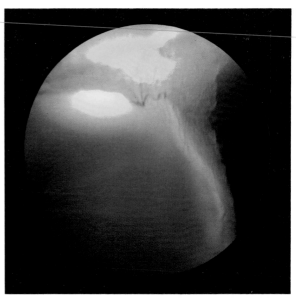

524 Retinal detachment (Shetland Sheepdog, 17 months old, sable) The appearance of total detachment through a dilated pupil.

525 Retinal detachment (Shetland Sheepdog, 9 months old, tricolour) Detachment and disinsertion.

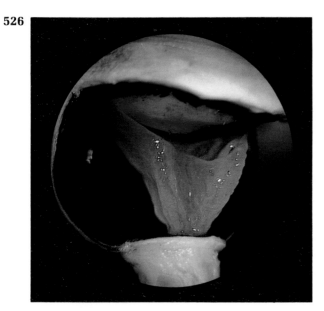

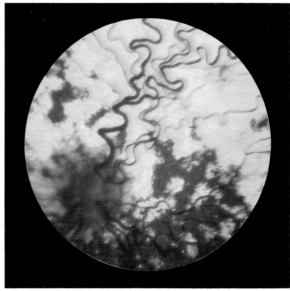

526 Retinal detachment (Rough Collie, 6 months old, tricolour) Detachment and disinsertion (post-mortem specimen).

527 Blood vessel tortuosity (Rough Collie, 6 months old, tricolour) Excessive vascular tortuosity—note coloboma of the disc.

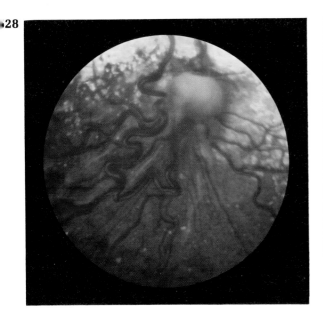

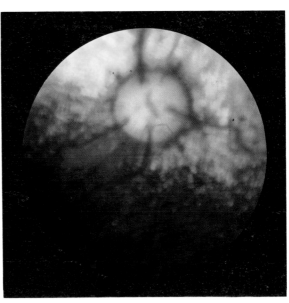

528 Blood vessel tortuosity (Rough Collie, 6 months old, tricolour) The other eye of the same dog—again note the excessive tortuosity and disc coloboma.

529 Vascular anomaly (Shetland Sheepdog, 3 years old, tricolour) Aberrant arteriolar loop at the edge of the disc at 7 o'clock, protruding forwards into the vitreous.

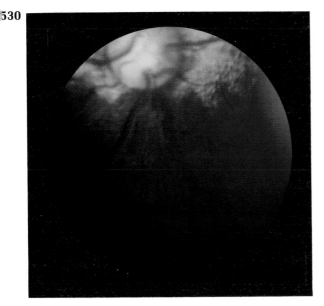

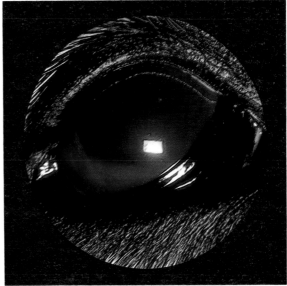

530 Vascular anomaly (Rough Collie, 7 weeks old, sable) Aneurysms on retinal blood vessels.

531 Hyphaema (Rough Collie, 18 months old, sable) Intraocular haemorrhage may be the presenting sign of collie eye anomaly.

Retinal Dysplasia

532

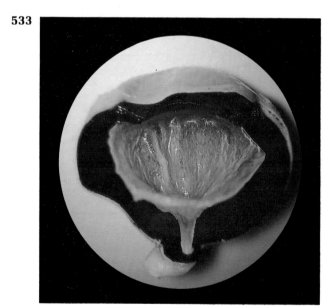

532 Sealyham, 8 weeks old The ophthalmoscopic appearance of total retinal detachment.

533

534

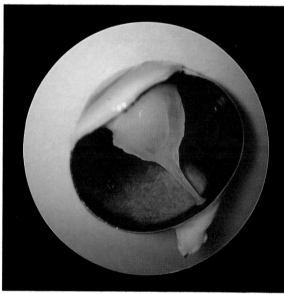

533 Sealyham, 4 months old Post-mortem specimen showing total infundibular-type detachment (lens removed).

534 Sealyham, 3 months old Similar to the previous figure showing funnel-shaped total detachment.

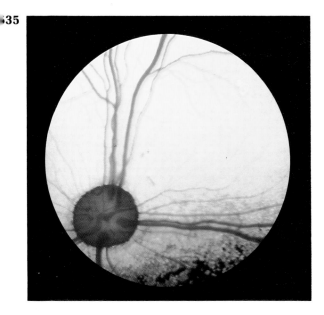

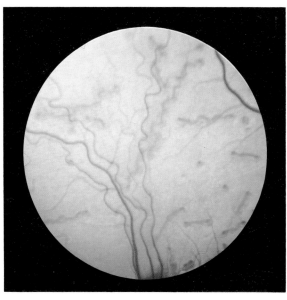

535 English Springer Spaniel, 9 months old
Multifocal retinal dysplasia. A very mild case with
two small retinal folds just beyond the disc edge at 2
o'clock.

536 English Springer Spaniel, 5 months old
Multifocal retinal dysplasia. Typical retinal folds in
a tapetal fundus superior to the disc.

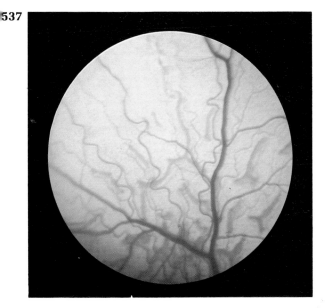

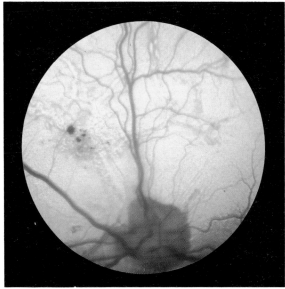

537 English Springer Spaniel, 6 months Similar but
more severe than the previous figure.

538 English Springer Spaniel, 15 months old In
addition to retinal folds also note areas of increased
reflectivity and pigmentation in the affected region.

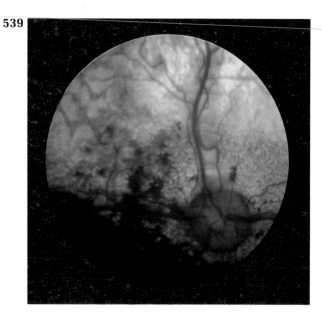

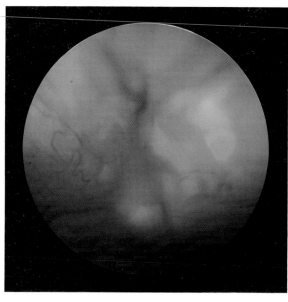

539 English Springer Spaniel, 2 years old More severe with some retinal detachment.

540 English Springer Spaniel, 5 months old Extensive detachment.

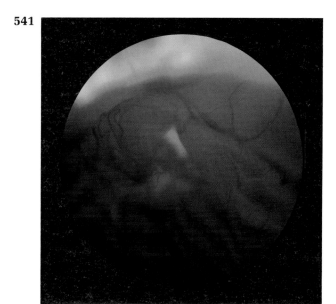

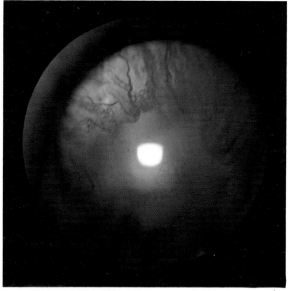

541 English Springer Spaniel, 18 months old Funnel-shaped total retinal detachment.

542 English Springer Spaniel, 8 months old Ophthalmoscopic appearance of infundibular detachment. Note the similarity to **532** in a Sealyham.

543 English Springer Spaniel, 5 months old
Post-mortem specimen showing total
infundibular-type detachment. Note the similarity
to Figures **533** and **534**.

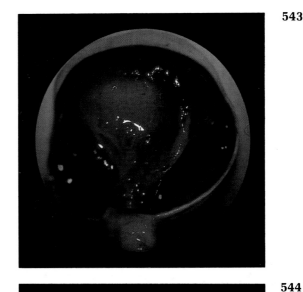

543

544 English Springer Spaniel, 7 weeks old Folds of
multifocal retinal dysplasia visible in the tapetal
fundus.

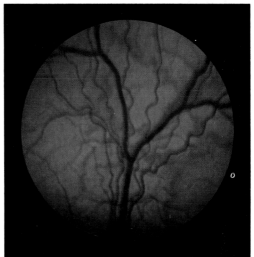

544

545 Cavalier King Charles Spaniel, 8 months old
Retinal folds in the typical position for multifocal
retinal dysplasia.

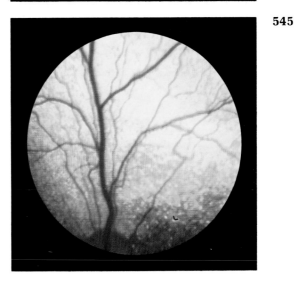

545

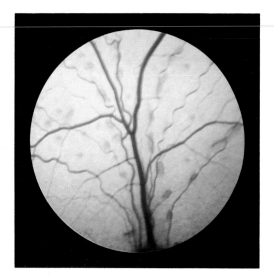

546 Three-quarter Golden Retriever x quarter Labrador Congenital and resembling hereditary multifocal forms in pure-bred dogs. Unknown aetiology.

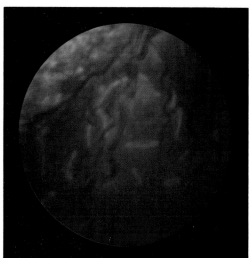

547 Rough Collie, 10 weeks old, tricolour Retinal folds in the non-tapetal fundus. Originally, and incorrectly, thought to be part of collie eye anomaly.

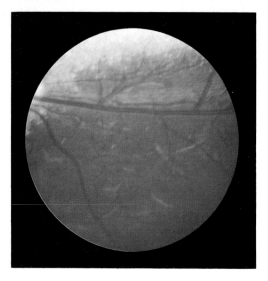

548 Beagle, 3 months old, tricolour Transient retinal folds in the non-tapetal fundus.

Other Retinopathies
The Dog

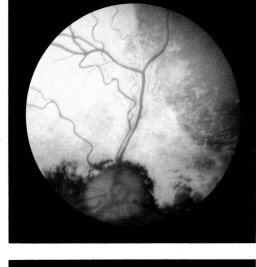

549 Post-inflammatory retinopathy (Sheepdog, 1 year old) Note the area of increased reflectivity, denoting retinal degeneration, in the upper right quadrant.

550 Post-inflammatory retinopathy (Labrador, 8 years old) Increased reflectivity in the tapetal region, together with some pigmentary disturbance in the lower left quadrant adjacent to the optic disc.

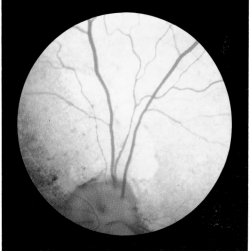

551 Post-inflammatory retinopathy (Greyhound, 2 years old) Generalised but patchy increased reflectivity with early changes of optic atrophy. This dog was unvaccinated and others in the litter were affected with retinal degeneration.

552 Post-inflammatory retinopathy (Labrador, 5 years old) Generalised retinal degeneration but note the change in tapetal colour from green to gold in the more severely affected parts.

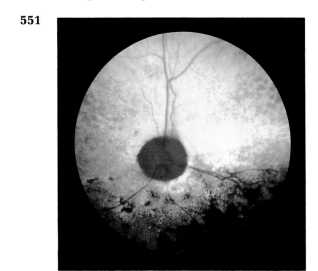

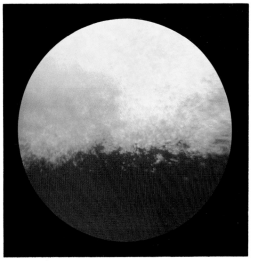

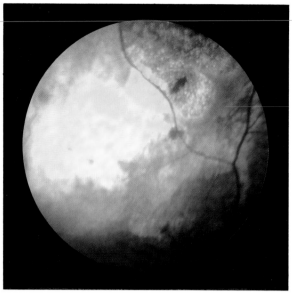

553 Post-inflammatory retinopathy (Border Collie, 13 years old, blue merle) The focal area of retinal degeneration is lateral to the disc. The other eye of this dog had a generalised retinopathy.

554 Post-inflammatory retinopathy (German Shepherd Dog, 7 years old) Typical changes of increased reflectivity and abnormal pigmentation. The other eye of this dog was normal.

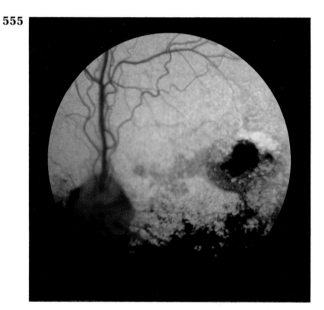

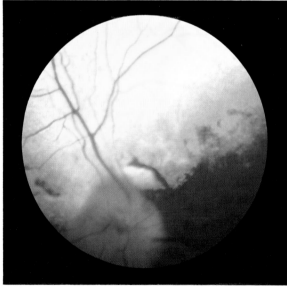

555 Post-inflammatory retinopathy (Sheepdog, 6 years old) Chorioretinitis with heavy pigmentation in the centre of the lesion.

556 Post-inflammatory retinopathy (Crossbred, 1 year old) Abnormal reflectivity and pigmentation. This dog was known to have had canine distemper.

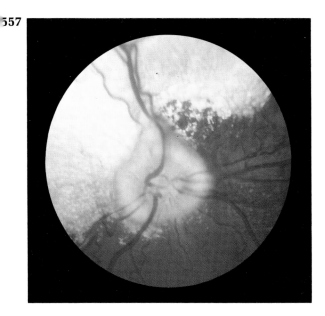

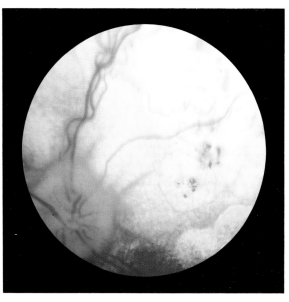

557 Post-inflammatory retinopathy (Crossbred, 6 years old) Peripapillary lesion on the medial side of the disc.

558 Post-inflammatory retinopathy (Crossbred, 6 years old) Other eye of dog in previous figure showing more extensive areas of retinal degeneration and demonstrating asymmetry of the two eyes. This dog was known to have had pyrexia and fits at a younger age and the lesions in both eyes were non-progressive over several years.

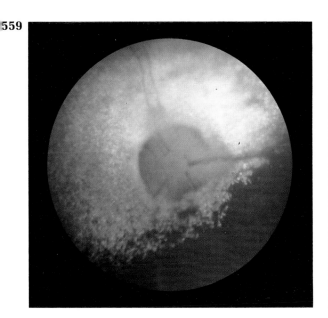

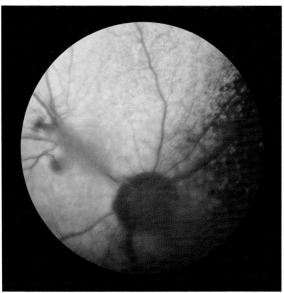

559 Post-inflammatory retinopathy (Dobermann, 8 years old) Advanced and severe retinal degeneration and optic atrophy.

560 Post-inflammatory retinopathy (English Springer Spaniel, 3 years old) Note the exudate and neovascularisation.

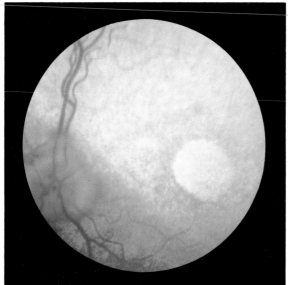

561 Post-inflammatory retinopathy (Labrador, 10 years old) Pigmentary retinopathy but note the difference to central progressive retinal atrophy (PRA).

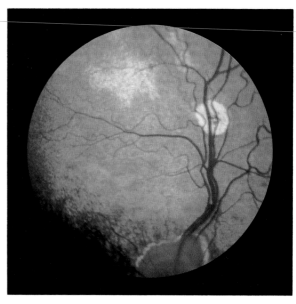

562 Post-inflammatory retinopathy (Labrador, 8 years old) Another pigmentary retinopathy with areas of increased reflectivity and unlike central PRA.

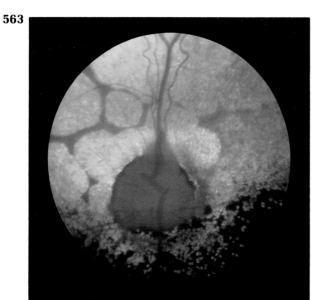

563 Post-inflammatory retinopathy (Afghan Hound, 5 years old) Another pigmentary retinopathy.

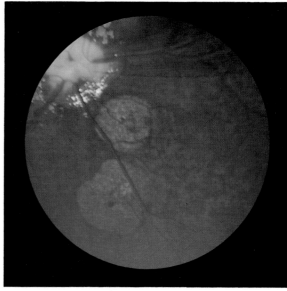

564 Post-inflammatory retinopathy (Greyhound, 18 months old) Focal areas of depigmentation in the non-tapetal fundus.

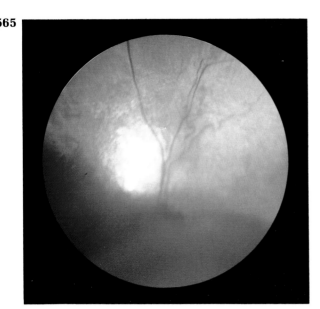

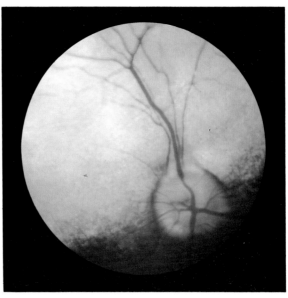

565 Retinal degeneration (Smooth-haired Fox Terrier, 7 years old) Retinopathy due to glaucoma—note the dislocated lens in the lower part of the photograph.

566 Retinal degeneration (Whippet, 8 years old) 'Sudden acquired retinal degeneration (SARD)'—note the early reflectivity visible in the tapetal region. This dog was presented with sudden blindness and with no changes in the fundus appearance until a subsequent examination.

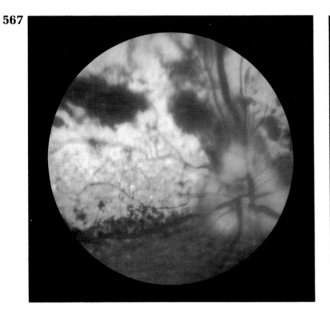

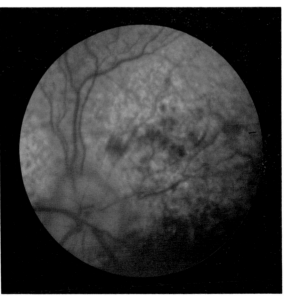

567 Retinal haemorrhage (Crossbred, 6 years old) Hypertensive retinopathy with renal disease.

568 Retinal haemorrhage (Standard Poodle, 8 years old) Diabetic retinopathy—diabetes of several years' duration.

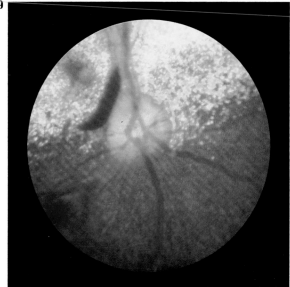

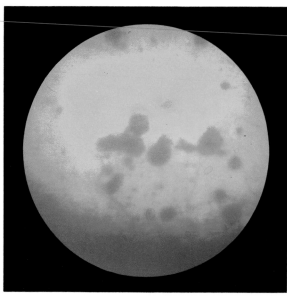

569 Retinal haemorrhage (Cocker Spaniel, 6 years old) Warfarin poisoning—note the retinal haemorrhage and anaemia of the retinal vessels.

570 Retinal haemorrhage (Crossbred, 13 years old) Retinal haemorrhages in a case of generalised lymphosarcoma.

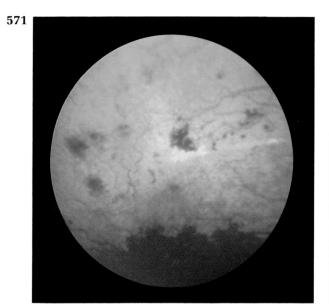

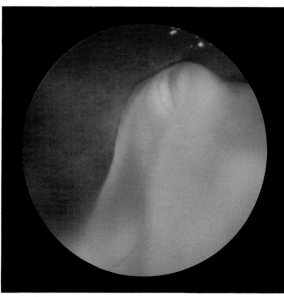

571 Retinal haemorrhage (Labrador, 12 years old) Multiple retinal haemorrhages in an aged dog.

572 Retinal detachment (Miniature Poodle, 4 years old) Total retinal detachment in both eyes. Unknown aetiology.

573 Retinal detachment (Crossbred, 7 years old)
Serous or exudative retinal detachment with blisters
of detached retina (appearance through the pupil).

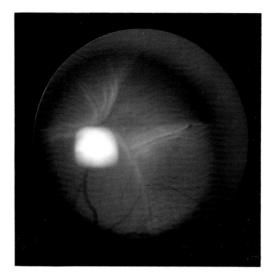

574 Retinal detachment (Crossbred, 9 years old)
Serous retinal detachment.

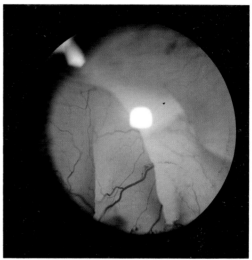

575 Coloboma (Beagle, 14 months old) Atypical
coloboma of the retina and choroid—both eyes are
affected but asymmetrically.

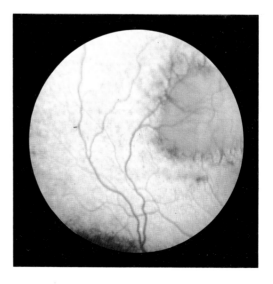

576 Progressive retinal atrophy (Abyssinian, 6 months old) Rod-cone dysplasia. Hereditary and due to a dominant gene.

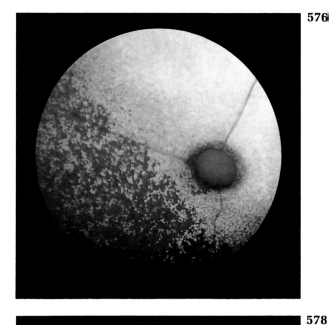

576

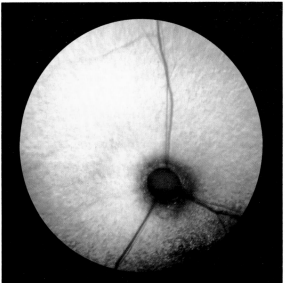

577

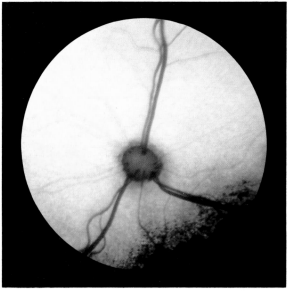

578

577 Progressive retinal atrophy (Abyssinian cross, 6 months old) Note the increased tapetal reflectivity and attenuated retinal blood vessels.

578 Normal fundus (Abyssinian cross, 6 months old) Littermate to the animal shown in the previous figure, showing normal tapetal reflectivity and normal retinal blood vessels.

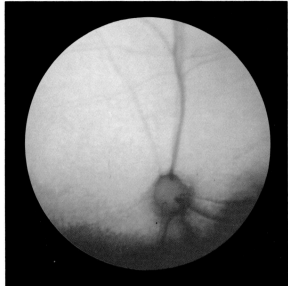

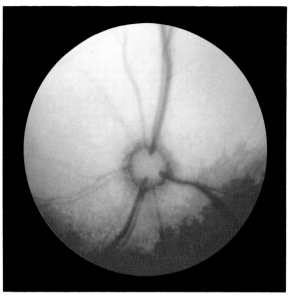

579 Progressive retinal atrophy (Abyssinian cross, 10 weeks old) Early changes.

580 Normal fundus (Abyssinian cross, 10 weeks old) Normal littermate control.

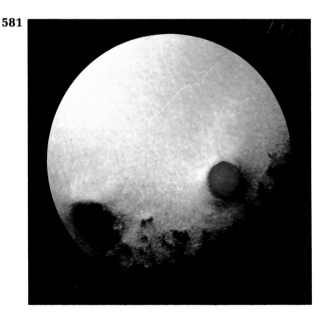

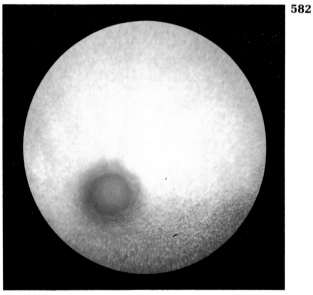

581 Progressive retinal atrophy (Abyssinian cross, 12 months old) Advanced retinal degeneration. Note tapetal degeneration in the area centralis region. Same cat as **579**.

582 Progressive retinal atrophy (Siamese, 4 years old) Bilateral, symmetrical and of possible hereditary origin.

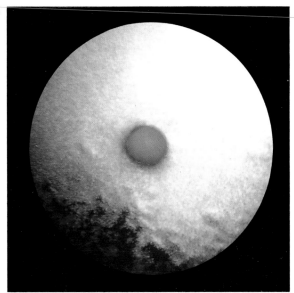

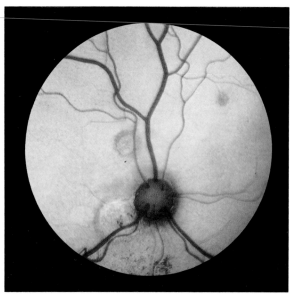

583 Retinal degeneration (DSH tabby and white, 3 years old) Advanced retinal degeneration with ghost vessels. Unknown aetiology.

584 Focal retinal degeneration (DSH, 5 years old) Several areas of focal retinal degeneration. The aetiology is probably toxoplasmosis.

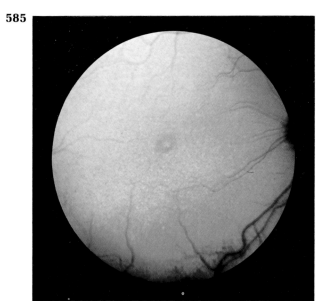

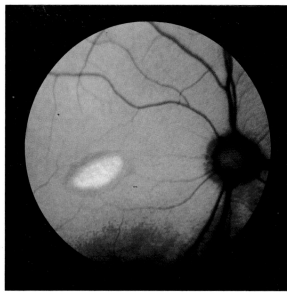

585 Taurine retinopathy (Experimental-DSH) Note early small focal spot at the area centralis immediately lateral to the optic disc.

586 Taurine retinopathy (Experimental-DSH) Larger, oval reflective area.

587 Taurine retinopathy (Experimental-DSH) Area of retinal degeneration now approaching the optic disc.

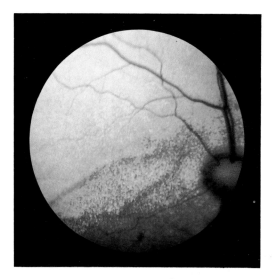

588 Taurine retinopathy (Experimental DSH) Two areas of retinal degeneration have now met in a bridge immediately superior to the optic disc.

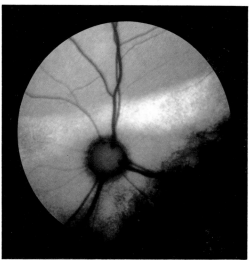

589 Taurine retinopathy (Experimental DSH) Generalised retinal degeneration—advanced case.

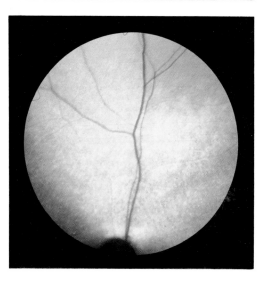

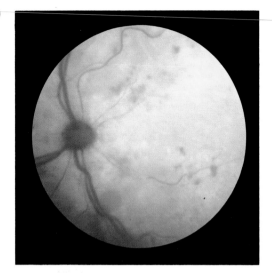

590 Renal retinopathy (DSH, 12 years old) Retinal haemorrhages, exudates and detachment.

591

591 Renal retinopathy (DSH, 13 years old) Serous retinal detachment.

592

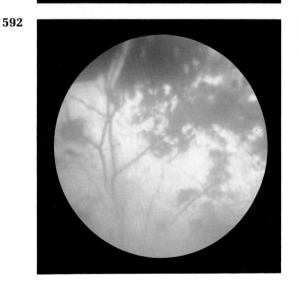

592 Diabetic retinopathy (DSH, 15 years old) Multiple retinal haemorrhages following prolonged administration (6 years) of megestrol acetate.

593 Diabetic retinopathy (DSH, 10 years old)
Retinal haemorrhages and detachment visible
through the pupil. Similar aetiology to the condition
shown in the previous figure (8 years'
administration of megestrol acetate).

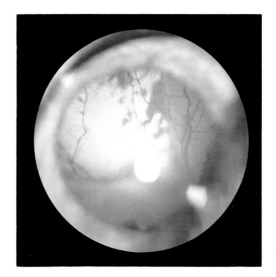

594 Retinal haemorrhage (DSH, 10 years old)
Haemorrhage following trauma.

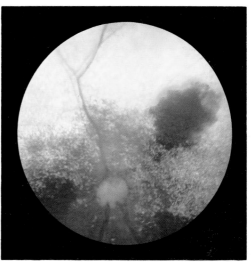

595 Retinal detachment (DSH, 4 months old) Total
detachment, both eyes—note the central hole in the
retina. Probably a congenital anomaly.

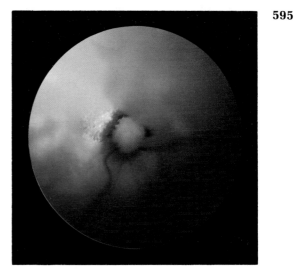

596

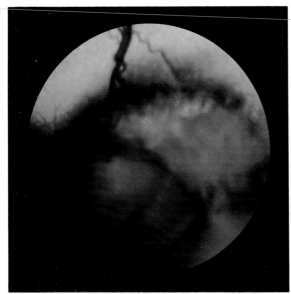

596 Coloboma (DSH, 12 months old) Colobomata affecting the retina, choroid and optic disc.

The Horse

597

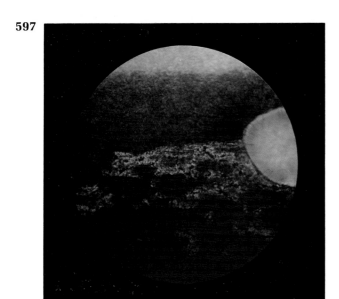

598

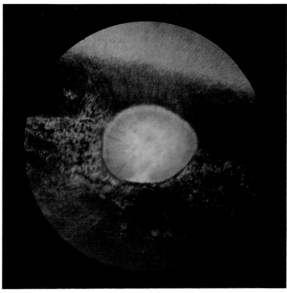

597 Retinopathy (Hunter-type, 7 years old)
Peripapillary retinal degeneration.

598 Retinopathy (Hunter-type, 7 years old)
Peripapillary retinopathy on both sides of the disc.

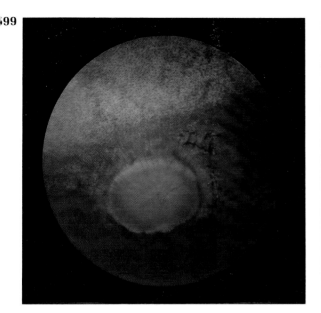

599 Retinopathy (pony, 25 years old, chestnut)
Peripapillary and pigmentary retinopathy.

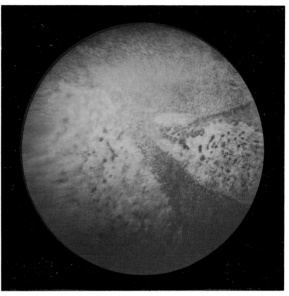

600 Retinopathy (Hunter-type, 12 years old, bay)
Partial retinopathy.

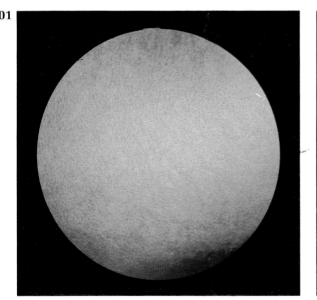

601 Retinopathy (Thoroughbred, yearling)
Generalised progressive retinal atrophy.

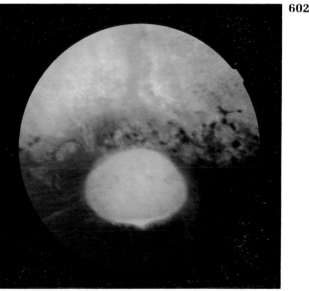

602 Retinal detachment (Hunter-type, 6 months old) Total detachment in both eyes—probably congenital.

603

604

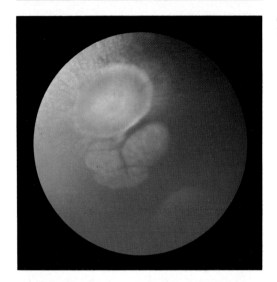

604 Coloboma (Thoroughbred, 2 months old) Retinal colobomata in the typical position.

605

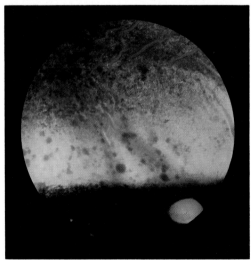

605 Retinal haemorrhage (Thoroughbred foal, a few days old) Multiple, small retinal haemorrhages in Convulsive Foal Syndrome (post-mortem specimen).

170

The Sheep

606 Retinal degeneration (Hill breed ewe) Bright blindness or primary toxic retinopathy due to the ingestion of bracken.

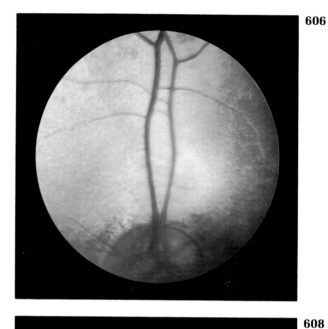

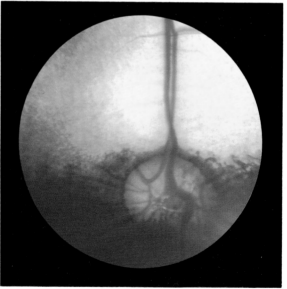

607 Retinal degeneration (Hill breed ewe) Note the attenuation of the retinal blood vessel. Aetiology as for **606**.

608 Retinal degeneration (Hill breed ewe) Note the increased tapetal reflectivity. Aetiology as for **606**.

The Optic Nerve

The final section on the optic nerve or optic disc which, with the retina, constitutes the ophthalmoscopic appearance of the fundus, should be studied closely with the previous section on the retina as in certain situations the two are difficult to divide. Illustrations showing the normal variations of the optic disc have been included in the previous section under each species.

Conditions of the canine optic nerve illustrated include papilloedema and optic neuritis which appear similar ophthalmoscopically and, with optic nerve tumour, increase the size of the optic disc.

Optic atrophy, optic disc cupping, and hypoplasia, all of which are illustrated, present as decreases in size of the optic disc. Two colobomata of the disc are shown in this section but to these should be added colobomata as seen in Collie Eye Anomaly, illustrated in **507** to **520**. In the horse optic atrophy is a condition which is not uncommon.

In cattle, papilloedema and consequent optic atrophy and retinal degeneration, as seen in cases of Vitamin A deficiency (**627–631**), are illustrated. Hereditary colobomata of the optic disc, of varying degrees of severity, are shown in the Charolais breed (**632–636**).

The Dog

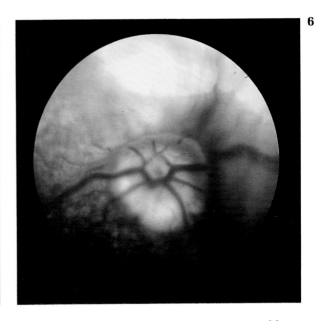

609 Papilloedema (West Highland White, 7 years old) Note the enlarged size of the disc and congestion of the retinal veins. The condition was bilateral and a pupillary light reflex was present.

610 Papilloedema (Miniature Poodle, 8 years old) Note the swollen disc protruding forwards.

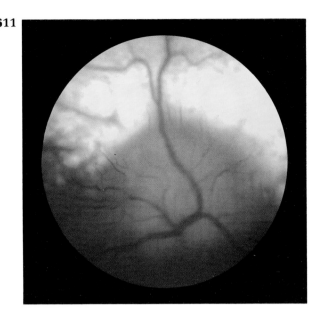

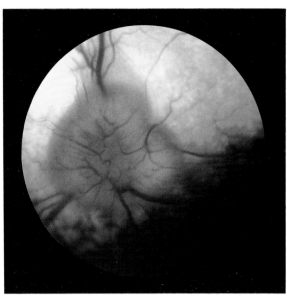

611 Optic neuritis (Maltese Terrier, 7 years old)
Presenting signs are sudden loss of vision and
absence of the pupillary light reflex. Note the similar
ophthalmoscopic appearance to papilloedema.

612 Optic neuritis (Labrador, 18 months old) The
other eye was affected but not as severely. This eye
showed optic atrophy months later.

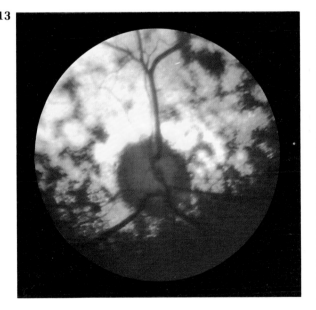

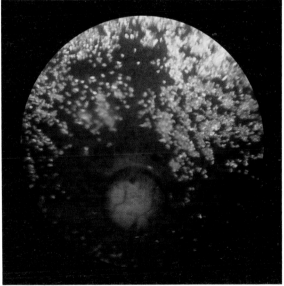

613 Optic atrophy (Border Collie, 5 years old)
Post-inflammatory optic nerve and retinal
degeneration of unknown aetiology.

614 Optic atrophy (Lhasa Apso, 18 months old)
Optic atrophy following prolapse of the globe.

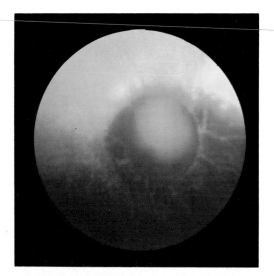

615 Optic disc cupping (Welsh Springer Spaniel female, 2 years old) Severe cupping following primary glaucoma.

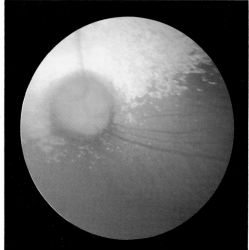

616 Optic disc cupping (English Springer Spaniel, 5 years old) Cupped disc together with retinal degeneration following primary glaucoma.

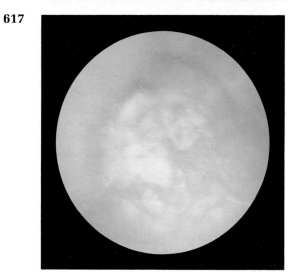

617 Optic nerve tumour (Miniature Poodle, 7 years old) Retrobulbar meningioma. Note also vitreal degeneration.

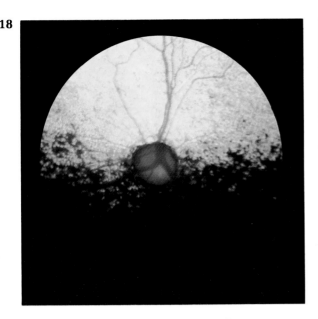 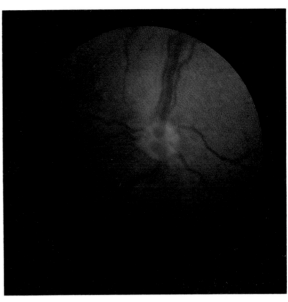

618 Optic nerve hypoplasia (Toy Poodle, 2 years old) Inherited in this breed. Compare this pathological condition with micropapilla in **396**.

619 Optic nerve hypoplasia (Shetland Sheepdog, 7 weeks old, sable) Unilateral in this case.

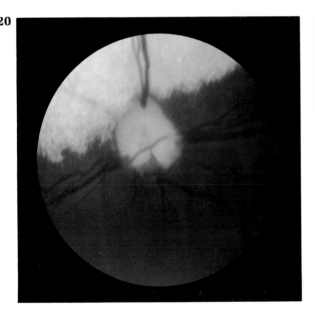 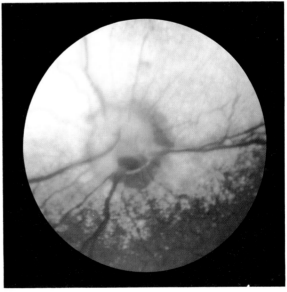

620 Coloboma (Basenji, 10 years old) Typical coloboma of the optic disc—inherited in this breed and associated with persistent pupillary membranes.

621 Coloboma (Beagle, 1 year old) Typical disc coloboma at 6 o'clock. Unilateral in this case with no evidence of heredity in this breed.

622

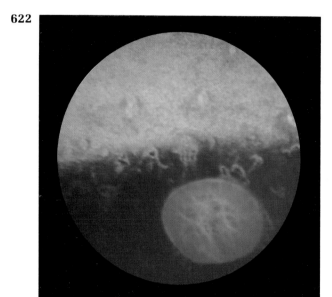

622 Optic atrophy (Thoroughbred, yearling)
Bilateral optic atrophy with secondary retinal
degeneration.

623

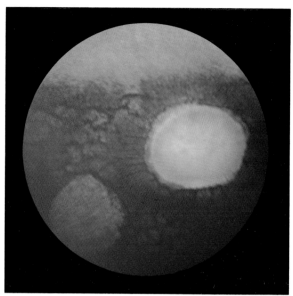

**623 Optic atrophy (Thoroughbred, 8 years old,
chestnut)** Optic atrophy and areas of retinal
degeneration.

624

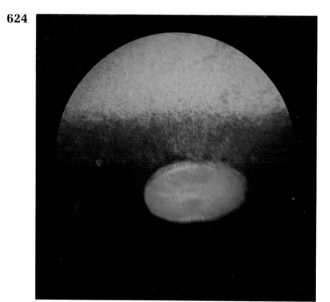

624 Optic atrophy (Welsh Cob, 5 years old) Note
the pale disc (the shape of the disc is not
significant).

625

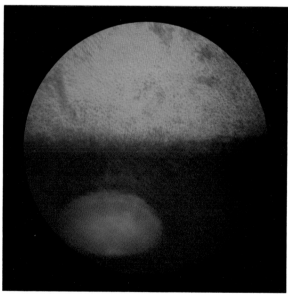

625 Normal (Welsh Cob, 5 years old) The other eye
of the same horse as shown in the previous figure, to
show the normal disc colour.

626 Optic nerve degeneration (Thoroughbred, 4 years old, bay) Proliferative lesion following a massive haemorrhage.

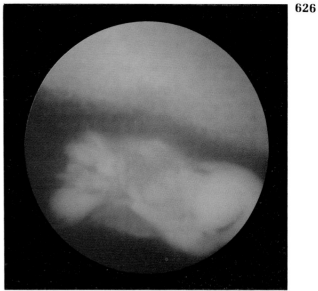

Cattle

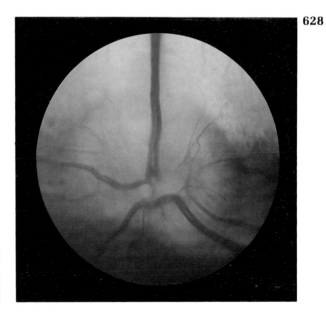

627 Papilloedema (Ayrshire calf) Papilloedema and small flame-shaped haemorrhage at 5 o'clock. Vitamin A deficiency.

628 Papilloedema (Shorthorn calf) Advanced papilloedema, caused by Vitamin A deficiency.

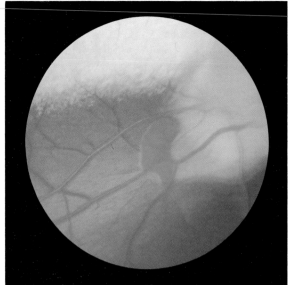

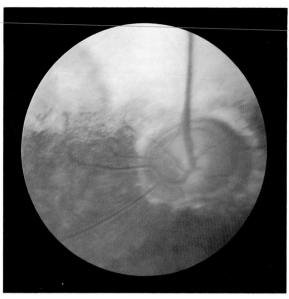

629 Papilloedema (Friesian bullock) Note the haemorrhage at the edge of the disc. Due to Vitamin A deficiency.

630 Optic atrophy (Shorthorn Heifer 18 months) Optic nerve degeneration following papilloedema. Vitamin A deficiency.

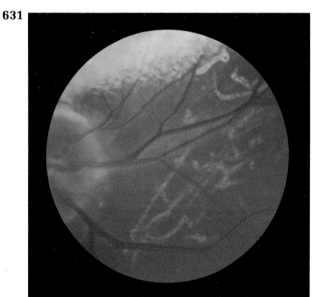

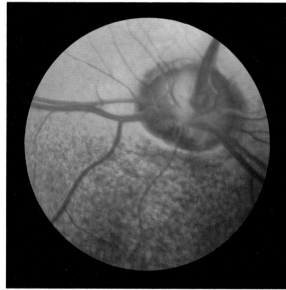

631 Retinal degeneration (Guernsey calf) Pale areas in a non-tapetal fundus. An advanced case of Vitamin A deficiency.

632 Coloboma (Charolais female, 2 years old) Mild colobomatous change with pigmentary disturbance in the non-tapetal fundus below the disc.

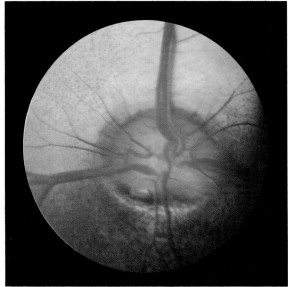

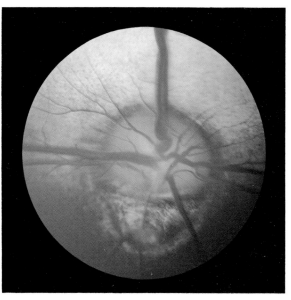

633 Coloboma (Charolais male) Slight coloboma at the lower edge of the disc.

634 Coloboma (Charolais male) Triangular coloboma immediately below the disc.

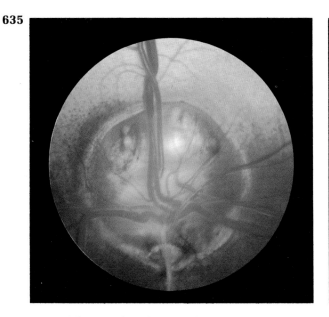

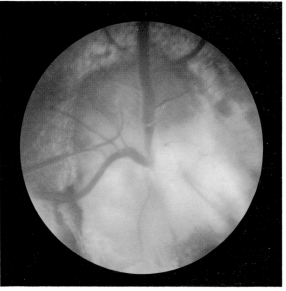

635 Coloboma (Charolais female 4 months) Coloboma of the whole disc and peripapillary region. Note the abnormal and persistent hyaloid artery.

636 Coloboma (Charolais bull) Severe coloboma of the disc and surrounding area.

Index

Numbers refer to figure numbers

Species Index

Index of Conditions

Index of Dog Breeds